# Dosage Calculations

*A Workbook with 120 Questions and Full Solutions For Nurses, Pharmacy Technicians and Other Medical Practitioners (Calculate Dosages With and Without Formulas)*

Published by Newstone Publishing

ISBN 978-1-989726-08-2 (paperback)

# Table of Contents

**Introduction and Disclaimer**................................................................ 15

**Chapter 1: Importance of Math in Medicine** .............................. 16

How Calculations Feature in Prescriptions ............................................ 16

Decrease of Body Medication in a Geometric Sequence .......................... 21

Illustration: Geometric Sequence in Medicine Decline ........................... 21

About Ratios & Proportions.................................................................. 22

**Chapter 2: About the Medication Order**.................................... 24

Processing & Utilization of MAR.......................................................... 24

Fundamental Parts of a Medication order ............................................. 26

**Chapter 3: Errors Associated with Medication Dosing**........... 29

Meaning and Implications of a Medication Error .................................... 29

Dosing Errors Common with Nurses .................................................... 30

Seriousness of Dosing Errors in the US ................................................ 30

Evidence of Effort to Reduce Dosing Errors ......................................... 31

Exact Measures taken by FDA to Minimize Medication Errors ............... 31

Specific Aspects of Drugs Reviewed by FDA ........................................ 31

FDA's Recommendations in the 2016 Guidelines .................................. 33

**Chapter 4: Math in the Field of Medicine**................................... 35

Importance of Math to the Physician..................................................... 35

Using Math to Maintain Patients' Health .............................................. 35

Using Math to Determine Suitable Prescription ..................................... 36

How Math is Helpful to Nurses............................................................ 36

General Use of Math in Dosage Calculations......................................... 36

Use of Math Skills to Convert Units between Varying Systems................ 37

Using Math in Calculation of Rates of IV Drip..................................................37

How Math Helps in Drug Titration ........................................................................37

Other Ways Competence in Math is Handy.........................................................37

How Pharmacists Make Use of Math Skills ..........................................................38

The Role of Math in Health Related Careers in General .................................38

Role of Math in Taking of Vital Signs...................................................................38

The General Role of Math in Dispensing Drugs ...............................................38

The Role of Math within the Operation Room..................................................39

How Math Helps in Effective Running of Health Facilities ............................39

**Chapter 5: Medication Dosing for Special Demographics ........................40**

Special Dosing for Children......................................................................................40

Why Children Respond Differently to Medication ...........................................41

Aspect of Oral Absorption........................................................................................41

Increase in Gastric pH ...............................................................................................41

Additional Factors Affecting Drug Absorption in Kids ...................................41

Drug Administration Route & Regime ..................................................................42

Manner of Writing a Prescription ..........................................................................43

Warning to Guardians of Kids .................................................................................43

About Dosage Calculations for Children ..............................................................44

Adverse Reactions to Medication ...........................................................................45

Importance of Reporting Adverse Reactions in Children ...............................45

Minding Home Safety for Children .......................................................................45

Special Dosing for the Elderly .................................................................................46

Why Medics Should Inquire About Use of Herbal Medication ....................47

How to Ascertain Quality in Prescribing for the Elderly.................................47

The Issue of Polypharmacy........................................................................47

Why Polypharmacy is a Concern ..............................................................48

Why the Elderly are more adversely impacted by Polypharmacy ...........48

Dosing Considerations Specific to the Elderly .......................................49

How to Tailor Adult Prescription to Suit the Elderly..............................50

Dosing Unsuitable for the Elderly ..........................................................51

The Importance of Beers Criteria ............................................................52

Ways of Improving Practices in Prescribing ...............................................53

Why Under-Dosing is also an Issue..........................................................53

Medication Affordability as an Issue .......................................................54

How to Prescribe for Expectant Patients .....................................................54

Medical Factors Unique to Pregnant Women...............................................55

The Choice to Make: Baby or Mother? ....................................................55

Factors to Consider in Prescribing for Expectant Mothers .........................56

Ease of Drug to Pass through the Fetus' Placenta....................................56

Mother's Gestational Stage........................................................................56

Physiological Effects of Medications during Pregnancy ..........................57

How Patient's Values Affect Treatment ........................................................58

Prescribing Considerations When the Mother Has Health Issues ...............59

How to Select Medication for Pregnant Patients ......................................60

How to Select Medication for Pregnant Patients ......................................62

**Chapter 6: Prescribing At the Time of Emergency ...................... 63**

Authority to Prescribe in Non- emergency Situations..................................63

Prescribing Authority of a Physician across States......................................65

Prescribing Authority of Health Care Givers in an Emergency...................65

**Chapter 7: How to Interpret Medical Orders** .................................................**68**

Medical Abbreviations Commonly Used.................................................68

    Medication Related Abbreviations .................................................68

The Apothecary Abbreviation System .................................................81

    Weight & Volume Abbreviations .................................................81

    Abbreviations Relating to Administration of Medication.................................................82

    Abbreviations Discouraged in the Medical Field .................................................82

Roman Numerals in Medicine .................................................83

    Basic Roman Symbols.................................................84

    Repetition in Writing Roman Numerals .................................................84

    How to Write Massive Numbers as Roman Numerals .................................................85

    How to Write Very Big Numbers as Roman Numerals.................................................86

Rules Guiding Calculations Involving Roman Numerals .................................................86

    The Upper and Lower Case.................................................88

    About Fractions.................................................88

**Chapter 8: How to Interpret Drug Orders** .................................................**89**

A Table Useful in Dosage Conversions.................................................89

Abbreviated Doctor's Orders Exemplified .................................................90

Abbreviations Specific to Medication Administration Frequency .................................................91

    Understanding the PRN.................................................92

How to Tackle Dosage Problems.................................................92

    How to Convert Dosing Units involving Mass .................................................93

    Illustration: Conversion of Micrograms to Milligrams.................................................93

    Illustration: Conversion of Pounds to Kilograms.................................................93

    How to Convert Dosing Units involving Volume .................................................93

Illustration: Conversion of Liters to Microliters ................................................. 94

How to Convert Dosing Units involving Time ............................................... 94

How to Convert Dosing Units Involving Mass ............................................. 94

Illustration: Calculation of Tablets when Mass Ordered differs from Available ...... 94

Illustration on Calculation on No. of Tablets to Dispense ........................... 95

How to Convert Dosing Units involving Mass vs Liquid ............................ 95

Illustration: Calculation of Drug Proportion to Administer from Available ........... 96

Illustration to Calculate Medication Dose to Administer per IV Infusion .............. 96

Crucial Terms & Abbreviations relating to IV Medication Administration ................. 97

Illustration to Decipher Doctor's Prescription ............................................. 98

Determining Content in IV Fluids ..................................................................... 98

How to Calculate Mass when provided with volume and dosage ........................... 98

Illustration to Calculate Dextrose Concentration in a Fluid .................................. 98

How to Calculate the Rate of IV Flow given Volume and Period ............................. 99

Illustration: Calculation of Infusion Flow Rate Given Volume & Time .................. 100

Calculations Involving Volume, Time & Rate of IV Drop ...................................... 100

Illustration: Calculation of IV Flow Rate Given Drop factor & Time ..................... 100

Illustration: Calculation of IV Flow Rate given Drug & Drop Factor ..................... 101

Calculations Involving Maintenance of Fluid ..................................................... 102

Illustration: Calculation of Infant's Fluid Requirement Given Weight .................. 102

Illustration: Calculation of Infant's Best IV Flow Rate ........................................ 103

Illustration: Calculating Appropriate Fluid Flow Rate Given Volume & Time ...... 103

Calculations Involving Weight Based Dosage ....................................................... 104

Dosage Formula Given Weight ........................................................................... 104

Illustration to Determine if Dr's Dosage is Within Suitable Range ...................... 104

Illustration on Calculation of Dosage in mL ......................................................... 105

Calculations Involving Mass over Time & IV Rate ....................................................... 106

Illustration on Calculation of Infusion Flow Rate in mL/hr................................... 106

Illustration on Calculation of Infusion Pump Flow Rate ....................................... 107

Why there is Great Potential in the Nursing Career ..................................................... 109

The Certified Nursing Assistant ............................................................................... 110

The Invaluable School Nurse..................................................................................... 110

Nurses Specializing in Handling HIV/AIDS ........................................................... 110

The Radiology Nurse................................................................................................... 110

Nurses within the American Red Cross................................................................... 111

The Public Health Nurse............................................................................................ 111

Nurses Specialized in Nutrition and Fitness ......................................................... 111

The Oncology Nurse................................................................................................... 111

Nurses Specialized in Neonatal Intensive Care Unit ........................................... 111

Nurse Handling Plastic Surgery .............................................................................. 112

Nurses working within Prisons & Other Correction Facilities............................ 112

Nurses Charged with Rehabilitation ....................................................................... 112

Nurses Handling Labor & Delivery ......................................................................... 113

Nurses Handling Burns ............................................................................................. 113

The Invaluable Surgical Nurses................................................................................ 113

Nurses for Pediatric Home Care............................................................................... 114

The Forensic Nurse..................................................................................................... 114

The Geriatric Nurse .................................................................................................... 114

Nurses Providing Care in Rural Settings................................................................ 114

The ER Nurse............................................................................................................... 114

Nurses Providing Long-Term Care.................................................................115

Nurses of the Intensive Care Unit ...............................................................115

The Pediatric Nurse .....................................................................................115

The Hospice Care Nurse ..............................................................................115

Nurses Handling Telephonic Triage.............................................................116

Opportunities of a Nurse Educator .............................................................116

Opportunities for an Epidemics Research Nurse.........................................116

Opportunities for a Dialysis Nurse .............................................................117

Opportunities for a Bioterrorism Nurse .....................................................117

Important Role of Senior Home Care Nurse................................................117

Opportunities for Legal Nurse Consultant .................................................117

Opportunities for the Pharmaceutical Research Nurse ..............................118

Interesting Opportunities for the Flight Transport Nurse..........................118

Opportunities for the Occupational Health Nurse......................................118

Adventures of a Cruise Ship Nurse.............................................................118

Management Role of the Charge Nurse........................................................118

Opportunities for the Wound Ostomy Continence Nurse ...........................119

Opportunities for Nursing in Infusion Therapy..........................................119

Role of the Coordinating Transplant Nurse ...............................................119

Nursing Opportunities in Psychiatric Mental Health ................................119

How to Practice as a Family Nurse..............................................................120

Opportunities for Nursing in the Medical-Surgical Practice .....................120

Nursing Opportunities in the Control of Infectious Diseases.....................120

Nursing Opportunities in Health Administration.......................................120

Nursing Role in Disaster Management ........................................................120

Interesting Role as a Travel Nurse ...................................................121

Role of a Nursing Practitioner .........................................................121

Role of the Nursing Anesthetist........................................................121

Role of the Certified Nurse Midwife ..................................................121

Role of the Neonatal Nurse Practitioner ...........................................121

**Chapter 9: Dosing Math for the Pharmacist ........................................... 123**

The Role of Clinical Pharmacists in Linking Patients and Physicians ...................... 124

Importance of Clinical Pharmacists in different Departments ................................. 125

Hospital Pharmacists vs Clinical Pharmacists.................................................127

Importance of Clinical Pharmacists .................................................................127

The Role of Clinical Pharmacists.................................................................... 128

How Clinical Pharmacists Ensure Proper Care for Patients................................. 129

Where to Find Clinical Pharmacists ............................................................... 129

Calculation Methods Involving Ratios & Proportions ..................................... 130

Illustration on Ratio/Proportion Working.................................................... 130

Illustration on how to Turn ratio into Fraction............................................131

Calculation Methods Involving Dimensional Analysis.................................... 131

Illustration of Dimensional Analysis (DA) ................................................... 132

Dosing Calculations for Liquids and Solids.................................................. 132

Appropriate Formula in Dilution of Medications .......................................... 133

Illustration involving Dilution of Liquid Medication...................................... 133

Illustration to Calculate Concentration Level .............................................. 134

Illustration on Dilution of Medication Solids ............................................... 135

Illustration to Find Out Concentration .................................................... 136

Aliquot as a Measure ..............................................................................137

Illustration on Using the Aliquot............................................................137

Illustration on Using the Aliquot............................................................138

Alligation as a Measurement Method ......................................................139

**Chapter 10: Proper Medication Administration ........................... 140**

Various Routes of Administering Medication............................................140

Techniques of Medication Administration ................................................141

    Importance of Dosage and Dispensing Timing....................................141

    Need to Express Potential for Drug Problems ....................................142

Subcutaneous Injection ..........................................................................143

Buccal and Sublingual Medication Administration....................................144

    Benefits of Buccal and Sublingual Drug Administration .....................145

    Disadvantages of Buccal and Sublingual Drug Administration............145

The Transdermal Patch ...........................................................................145

About Intravenous Medication Administration..........................................145

Uses of IV medications ...........................................................................146

About standard IV lines...........................................................................146

    IV Infusion ......................................................................................147

    Drip infusion ...................................................................................147

    Pump infusion.................................................................................147

    IV Push...........................................................................................147

Types Of Central Venous Catheters.........................................................148

    Tunneled catheter ...........................................................................148

    (PICC) Peripherally inserted central catheter ...................................148

    Implanted Port................................................................................148

Drugs Typically Given By IV....................................................................148

Possible IV Side effects ............................................................ 149

    Injury to vessels of the blood or Site of injection ................................. 149

    Chances of Air embolism ........................................................ 149

    Potential for Blood clots ....................................................... 150

    Possibility of Infection ......................................................... 150

About Intravenous Fluid Regulation ............................................. 150

Importance Of IV Fluid Regulation .............................................. 150

    Infection Treatment Using Antibiotics ........................................ 151

Various Kinds Of Intravenous Fluid Regulation ................................ 151

    Electric pump regulation ...................................................... 151

    Manual regulation ............................................................ 151

What To Expect As Procedure Is Undertaken .................................. 151

Possible complications of IV fluid regulation ................................... 152

Use of the Infusion Pump ......................................................... 152

About Lactated Ringers ........................................................... 154

9% Normal Saline ................................................................. 154

5% Dextrose in Water ............................................................. 154

45% Normal Saline ................................................................ 155

About the Intravenous Intermittent Infusion ................................... 155

Guidelines For The Intravenous Fluid Therapy ................................. 156

    Routine maintenance .......................................................... 156

    Fluid resuscitation ............................................................ 156

    Redistribution ................................................................ 156

    Replacement .................................................................. 157

Set Procedures for prescribing Fluids ........................................... 157

The Intramuscular Injection ............................................................................ 158

    Targeting the Arm's Deltoid Muscle............................................................ 158

    Vastus Lateralis Muscle of the thigh........................................................... 158

    Ventrogluteal Muscle of the hip.................................................................. 158

    Dorsogluteal Muscle of the buttocks .......................................................... 158

The Drip Bar of Modern Day.......................................................................... 159

    Interesting Trend Developing – IVs on demand.......................................... 159

    Reasons Why People May Wish for IVs ...................................................... 160

**Practice Questions** ........................................................................... **162**

**Answers to Practice Questions** ....................................................... **186**

# Introduction and Disclaimer

This book is designed to provide detailed information regarding dosage calculations in the workplace and how to effectively go about determining the right dosage amounts. A series of practice questions is included in the second half of this book, along with full solutions. Great care must be taken when calculating dosages because incorrect dosages can harm patients. The author, publisher or this book will not be held liable for any incorrect calculations or mistakes that practitioners make as a result of using this book. Each practitioner should do their due diligence to ensure administered dosages are correct.

# Chapter 1: Importance of Math in Medicine

Medical practitioners, be they physicians or nurses, face situations that require the use of math, and this is something that they anticipate on a daily basis. For example, when there is need to write a prescription or to dispense medicine, math is involved. There are even cases where professionals in the medical field need to work or make presentations with graphs, and use of math here is inevitable. A good example is when research findings are being reported and there is need to show statistics in form of graphs, or instances where varying rates of success are being shown with respect to specific treatments.

You will also find math being utilized in X-rays, CAT scans and several other medical procedures. In general, numbers are made use of severally by medical practitioners, as they are handy at providing useful information, either for diagnostic or treatment purposes. When it comes to treatment, physicians, nurses, anesthetists and various other medical personnel cannot avoid using math either when prescribing medicine or dispensing it. The dosage must be right to the smallest measure, failure of which can lead to dire consequences on the part of the patient's health.

Gladly, medics are normally well trained in the area of dosage calculations, and even nurses who often administer day-to-day medications to patients have to pass tests related to dosage calculations. Also, nurses who are already practicing and other professionals in the medical field can now take advantage of books such as this one on dosage calculations, as it helps them refresh their memories and keep up to date with the best way to go about calculating doses of patients' medicine. Another group that will certainly find a book such as this helpful is that of aspiring nurses, and with the solved practice questions incorporated, the trainees are bound to find it easy to pass the exam part on dosage calculations.

### *How Calculations Feature in Prescriptions*

Calculations are a basic feature as far as prescribing of medicine is concerned, as every prescription doctors write has a measure commensurate with the seriousness of the patient's illness, the age of the patient, sometimes the patient's weight, and such other aspects relating to the patient. You can expect a given prescription to have at least the actual name of the medicine being recommended for the patient as well as the dosage amount recommended.

In many cases, medications come from the manufacturing pharmaceuticals with guidelines showing the amount of medicine a patient of a certain weight should receive for a given illness, which is indicated in terms of mg per kg or milligrams per kilogram. It is then the doctor's duty to decide the number of milligrams of a particular medicine a particular patient should receive depending on the patient's weight. In case the medicine guidelines have their units as pounds and the daily parlance is in kilograms, the doctor ought to convert the given pounds to kilograms. That calls for capacity to do quick conversion calculations. It means the doctor needs to know how many kilograms a patient would weigh, given the patient's weight in pounds. The doctor would then need to calculate the amount of medicine in milligrams that the patient would need and then put that in the patient's prescription.

The doctor must also perform the task of determining the duration it should take for the patient to finish taking the prescribed amount of medicine. In there is a case of a patient requiring a prescription of one tablet per day and there is a bottle of 30 tablets to be given, those tablets should take a complete 30-day month to be finished. The math involved here is:

If it takes one day to consume one tablet, how many days will it take to consume 30 tablets? In other words, if 1 day matches 1 tablet, how many days will match 30 tablets?

It is simply 1 day/1 tablet x 30 tablets like this:

1 day/1 tablet x 30 tablets

From the above fraction, you can cancel out '1 tablet', which is the denominator, and when you cancel the 30 tablets as the matching numerator, what you get at the top is 30; the tablets having cancelled out. Essentially what will remain is 1 day x 30, which is 30 days.

In case the prescription required the patient to take three tablets in a day, the same bottle of tablets would take the patient 10 days to finish. The math involved will be as shown here below.

If it takes one day to consume 3 tablets, say 1 tablet three times in one day, how many days will it take to consume 30 tablets? In other words, if 1 day matches 3 tablets, how many days will match 30 tablets?

It is simply 1 day/3 tablets x 30 tablets like this:

1 day / 3 tablets x 30 tablets

In this instance, 3 tablets cancels out completely when gauged against the numerator of 30 tablets, and instead of 30 tablets you will now have 10. In short, what you will remain with is 1 day x 10, which works out to 10 days.

This helps the doctor or nurse in charge to determine the date of the next visit in case there is need for a review by the doctor immediately the prescribed medicine is finished.

A medical practitioner may also need to know the number of tablets a patient needs in case it is important for the patient to take one tablet twice a day for a week. Of course the number of tablets that would need to be prescribed is 14, and the math involved would look like this:

It is simply 2 tablets/1 day x 7 days like this:

2 tablets / 1 day x 7 days

1 day, which is the denominator, will cancel out completely, and the 7 days serving as the numerator will cancel to remain with only 7. Ultimately, the 2 tablets x 7 that remains will result to 14 tablets.

For ailments that need long-term management, patients may have a preference for prescriptions covering two or even probably three months, and it is only fair to have doctors and nurses well equipped with the appropriate dosage calculation skills. It is important that they be in a position to calculate with both speed as well as accuracy. Moreover, they need to do sufficient practice to enable them be able to make the calculations mentally, as opposed to making numerous references to a chart or books all day long.

There is also need for calculations from another angle, where doctors need to know the duration a given type of medicine remains in the patient's body. On the basis of this information, doctors can then decide the regularity with which that particular medicine needs to be administered, so as to ensure the patient's system always has an appropriate amount of medicine working. Needless to say, regulation of the number of times a given type of medicine is administered also serves to ensure the patient's system is not saturated with medicine in a dangerous manner.

Clearly, the mathematical absolute figures take up new meaning once used in the practice of medicine, and math in general turns out to be indispensable in this regard. Take an example where a doctor has prescribed medication to be taken every morning, and the dosage is 50mg every time. As would be expected, by the time the patient takes the second dose, the amount of medicine in the system will have gone down. For some medicines, the amount already washed out would have been higher than for others. Suppose for this particular medicine over 24hrs the body washes away 40% of the medicine taken in one dose. How much is that in terms of mg? It is certainly:

40/100 x 50mg

You can cancel out 50 versus 100, where 50 divided by 50 will be 1 and 100 divided by 50 will be 2. At this juncture, what you will be remaining with is:

40/2 x 1mg

The next step should be to cancel the numerator 40 against the denominator, 2, where 2 divided by 2 gives 1 and 40 divided by 2 gives 20. Finally what you will have is:

20/1 x 1mg

20 x 1mg = 20mg, and if you divide 20mg by the 1 below your 20mg will remain as it is because any number divided by 1 remains as it was before; no effect whatsoever.

So on the second morning of taking the dose of 50mg, the patient's body will have cleared 20mg of that first dose, and that means the patient's body will still be having some balance of that first dose of 50mg. The exact amount of medicine remaining will be 30mg, which is easy to confirm by calculating:

50mg − 20mg = 30mg

According to the doctor's prescription, the patient needs to take another dose of 50mg in the morning, which means the patient's body will now have more medicine than before. Exactly how much medicine will the patient's system have after the dosage on the second morning?

You can get the solution by adding the amount that you found remained in the body from the first dose to the newly administered dose. Simply put:

30mg + 50mg = 80mg

When making a prescription, the doctor takes into account what is expected to happen to the patient's body not only on Day 2 but also on Day 3, Day 4 and the days that follow, with regard to the amount of medicine in the body. So it is important to establish the amount of medicine still in the patient's body as the second day ends, to bring a new morning when the patient is expected to take another dose of 50mg. How much medicine will still be in the patient's body at this time? This is how to find out.

The amount at the beginning of Day 2 = 80mg

Amount washed off by the body = (40/100 x 80mg)

You can divide 80mg by 20 and the result will be 40mg, and to correspond to that division will be 100 divided by 20, which will give you 50. So at this point what you have is:

40/50 x 40mg

You can simplify the fraction by dividing 40 by 10 and 50 by 10, and what you will have is:

4/5 x 40mg

Certainly the denominator, 5 can cancel with 40mg, so that 5 divided by 5 gives 1 and 40mg divided by 5 gives 8mg. The amount of medicine the patient's body will have cleared out of the 80mg at the start of Day 2 is:

4/1 x 8mg = 32mg

Of great importance now is to find out how much medicine the body still retains before a fresh dose is given on Day 3. This is easy to find by subtracting the cleared amount from the starting amount as shown here below.

80mg – 32mg = 48mg

48mg of the particular medicine will still be in the patient's body.

As you get comfortable with such kind of calculations, or if you are already a numbers' person, you may wish to make your calculations shorter. For example, instead of seeking to establish the amount already washed out from the body and then subtracting the outcome from the original dose, you could delve straightaway into calculating how much medicine has been retained.

For example in the case of Day 2 where the patient started off with 80mg of medicine in the body, the amount retained is simply 60% of 80mg. After all, the amount that was washed off was 40% of 80mg. Let us see if the answer is the same as the one from the longer method.

60/100 x 80mg

Let us deal with the 60% first; and 60 divide by 20 produces 3 while 100 divided by 20 produces 5. So we now have:

3/5 x 80mg

We can now divide 5 by 5, which will give us 1 and then divide 80mg by 5, which produces 16mg. The fraction has now become:

3/1 x 16mg

We need to ignore the 1 as it has no impact on the fraction as a denominator, and then proceed to calculate 3 x 16mg.

3 x 16mg = 48mg.

So, just as in the longer method, this shorter one provides the important information that the patient's body still has 48mg of the particular medicine at the end of Day 2. Clearly, the amount of medicine in the patient's body at the beginning of a new day is increasing every time, and it is up to the doctor to decide the appropriate point to stop giving the body more medication. It is important to remember that much as it is important to retain sufficient amounts of medicine in the body, it is also crucial to guard against overdosing.

The information the doctor gets from calculations like the ones already shown helps to determine the period the patient should take the medicine or the duration to be covered by the prescription given. This may also explain one reason patients are weaned off some medications slowly by slowly in a gradual manner rather than having an abrupt end.

### Decrease of Body Medication in a Geometric Sequence

It is indisputable that medicine within the body continues to decrease as time passes, and the question medics consider of great importance is at what rate is the given medicine decreasing? The medicine could be clearing from the body at a rate of 10% per hour or any other rate depending on which medicine it is. Often this percentage is expressed in form of a rational number, so that the 10% is taken to be $\frac{1}{10}$. Whatever amount the patient had in the body at the beginning of any given hour, the amount decreases by $\frac{1}{10}$, and so at the end of that particular hour the amount of medicine remaining in the patient's body will be $\frac{9}{10}$ of the amount at the beginning of the hour.

Remember what happens in hour 1 is the same thing that happens in hour 2, hour 3 and so on, every time the end of the hour having the remaining medicine being $\frac{9}{10}$ of the amount that the patient had at the beginning of the hour. This development forms a sequence termed geometric sequence, which constitutes a decrease that is both rational and constant.

### Illustration: Geometric Sequence in Medicine Decline

Suppose a patient takes a tablet that contains 500mg of a given drug, and the rate of decline of the medicine is 10% per hour. The table here below shows the amount of drug remaining in the body at the end of every progressing hour.

| Hour | Mg. at the Start of the Hour | Mg at the End of the Hour |
|------|------------------------------|----------------------------|
| 1st Hour | 500 | 9/10x 500 = 450 |
| 2nd Hour | 450 | 9/10 x 450 = 405 |
| 3rd Hour | 405 | 9/10 x 405 = 364.5 |
| 4th Hour | 364.5 | 9/10 x 364.5 = 328.05 |
| ... | ... | ... |

This is the number sequence that the doctor considers in determining how regularly the patient should take the particular medicine being prescribed.

### *About Ratios & Proportions*

It is important for nurses to be competent in using ratios as well as proportions for the sake of administering medicines. They are expected to know the amount of medicine their patient requires relative to the patient's weight. They also need to be able to follow the orders given by the doctor.

It is important to note that prior to administration of any medicine to a patient, the person concerned, usually a nurse, has to read and comprehend the order of medication issued by the doctor. The next thing would be to calculate the particular dose the doctor will have written. One may wonder why the nurse needs to calculate the dose for the patient, but it is crucial to note that the doctor's order contains the medicine dose the patient requires in order to be cured, which may not necessarily match the dose on the medicine package. If the latter, known as the 'unit dose package' matches the dose ordered by the doctor, then there would be no need for the nurse to engage in fresh calculations.

Ordinarily, manufacturers of pharmaceutical drugs pack the medications in unit doses, and that often minimizes medical errors of either under or over dosing. However, there are several instances too where the manufacturers do not pre-package the medications according to the right unit doses, and so it is up to the respective hospital pharmacies to do the packaging once they receive the medications in bulk. One unit dose reflected on the packaging is equivalent to a single dosage.

In other instances, pharmaceutical manufacturers package medication just sufficient to take one patient through a period of 24 hours. It may be surprising that manufacturers could choose to package medications in 24hr doses, but hospitals find some benefits in such dosage packaging. For starters medications are generally protected as only the amount required within 24hrs is released from the pharmacy at a time, and bar-coding of such doses is easy. There are more benefits for this system, not least the fact that damaged medication packages are more easily noted.

On the overall, it is important for nurses and other medical staff dealing with medications to understand how dosing is done or even interpreted, as one is likely to require the skills at one time or the other if not always. In any case, there are instances where a patient's dosage, as per the doctor, may fall below the one indicated on the manufacturer's package, or even rise above it. In such a case, it would be necessary for the nurse to make dosing calculations for the patient. Before this important step can be successfully accomplished, the nurse, or whoever staff is concerned, must be adept at reading the doctors' medication order. For that reason, there are some things that need to be learnt first regarding doctors' medication orders.

# Chapter 2: About the Medication Order

By medication order is a prescription written by a doctor after diagnosing the patient with a particular ailment. For instance, a patient presenting at the doctor's with body temperature reaching 101°F and with the tonsils swollen, and in addition with some white patches appearing at the throat, may be diagnosed with strep throat. In such a case, the doctor would write the patient a prescription, which is the medication order, with details of the medications the patient needs to receive plus their respective doses. A medication order is also referred to some times as a physician's order.

For the sake of keeping up-to-date, it needs to be known that with computerization that has taken place even in the health sector, medication orders are being referred to differently, the name reflecting the fact that the orders or prescriptions are generated and transmitted electronically. A medication order created electronically is termed Computerized Practitioner Order Entry or CPOE. Other times it is referred to as Computerized Physician Order Entry or Computerized Provider Order Entry, but all in all the reference remains as CPOE. However, in some instances such a prescription goes by the reference, Computerized Provider Order Management or CPOM. The tendency to write prescriptions electronically is mostly found crucial by doctors for inpatients; those the doctors are seeing under hospitalization.

Being proficient at understanding the language of medication dosing is very important, and this importance can be understood when you consider there may be instances where the doctor has no time to enter the prescription into the computer, very likely in a case of emergency. In such cases, the doctor might issue the prescription verbally to the nurse. Sometimes the doctor might be away from the hospital premises but decides to issue the prescription on phone either to the nurse or hospital pharmacist because of the urgency of the situation. Both these members of staff need to be very clear what the medicine is that the doctor prescribed and also the exact dose the doctor said ought to be given to the patient for stabilization or to practically save the patient's life.

Certainly giving verbal medication orders is not the norm, and the doctor concerned is expected to write and sign a formal order later as per the institution's policy, which is likely to be within 24 hours.

***Processing & Utilization of MAR***

First of all it needs to be understood that when patients go to see a doctor, they have their good reasons pertaining to their ill health. Particularly they have symptoms that are indicators of something being wrong with their bodies, and these are, obviously, subjective. When being seen or assessed by the doctor, what is essentially being sought is data that is objective, and which is referred to as signs. The signs that the doctor observes help to make an appropriate medical diagnosis, and on the basis of this diagnosis the doctor designs a treatment plan for the patient.

For example, when a patient comes into the doctor's office or clinic complaining of sore throat, the discomfort in the sore throat is the symptom as expressed by the patient. When the doctor objectively assesses the patient and notices that the tonsils glands are swollen and there are white patches at the throat, these are the ones referred to in medical terms as signs. It is on the basis of these signs that the doctor makes an appropriate diagnosis and thereafter writes a prescription.

The doctor's prescription is then entered into a schedule meant to guide the medical staff in administering medication to the patient, which is referred to as the Medical Administration Record or MAR in short. Basically the information entered in the MAR comprises the medication given to the patient, the person who administered the medication and at what exact time. These days many hospitals are computerized and so the MAR is also in soft copy. It is, in fact, termed eMAR.

The action of the pharmacist entering the information provided in the medication order onto the computer system is described as 'taking off the order'. The nurse in charge of administering the medication looks at the information on eMAR and checks it against the corresponding medication order to ensure everything tallies. This process by the nurse is referred to as 'cosigning', and even in institutions where everything is done manually, there is normally a second nurse to verify that the information entered into the MAR is exactly as the doctor intended when writing the medication order.

Patients' safety is of paramount importance, and so irrespective of how small or big a health institution is, cosigning is taken seriously. At the same time, the doctor's order must always be complete with all the fundamental information, leaving no room for nurses, laboratory technicians or any other medical staff to speculate. A medication order basically comprises seven parts and the normal process ought not to continue if any of those parts is missing.

### Fundamental Parts of a Medication order

Medication should not particularly be administered on the basis of an incomplete medication order. Instead, the nurse should immediately get in touch with the concerned doctor for correction or completion of the medication order.

It ought to be noted that the nurse cannot purport to do the correct dosage calculations and to execute the medical order effectively if it is not even known what the information is that the doctor would have written on the medication order. So if a medical order is incomplete, it is rendered unusable until it is completed by the doctor. Of equal importance is the fact that a nurse or any other medical staff can be liable for prosecution for administering medication to a patient on the basis on an incomplete medication order.

There may be a case, for instance, where the doctor has prescribed Chloramphenicol for the treatment of an adult suffering from pneumonia but the medication order bears no dose, the doctor having inadvertently omitted it. Treatment for the patient should not proceed even where the nurse and the doctor have worked together for a long time and the nurse knows the doctor usually prescribed 1g to be administered intravenously every six hours for a whole seven days in medical cases like this. So, dose is a very crucial part of the medication order.

Another very important part of the medication order is the proper identification of the patient. In case patients' identification is not distinctively clear, there is the risk of the medication for different patients being mixed up, and a patient receiving the wrong medication can be disastrous. For that reason, a medication order must contain the patient's name in full, a unique number allocated to the patient, as well as the patient's birth date. For a patient who has been brought in on an emergency, the medical staff involved must ascertain that the information on the medication order corresponds to the particulars on the wrist band on the patient.

It is also required that the nurse inquires on her own the patient's name as well as the patient's birth date, just to be sure the medical record belongs to the correct patient. One ought to keep in mind that the medical record is the primary source of all other information pertaining to the patient's course of treatment, dosing included. Nurses are reminded of the importance of the patient's name and date of birth, and that a name is not sufficient on its own as two people within the same hospital ward or unit could have similar names. All other patient identifiers, inclusive of the number allocated the particular medical record, are secondary.

Another crucial part of a medication order is what is termed 'time stamp'. Which year and month and even day and time did the doctor write the medication order? The medication order must have all these specific details, and the dates indicated for administration of medication are no substitute.

A medication order also has a 'cutoff' for some kinds of medications, and this means the time the medical order should be deemed to have expired. Most commonly such expiration date is relevant when it comes to medications such as antibiotics, and the exact date is determined in reference to the starting period of medication administration. Often the starting point is the time of writing of the medical record, and the counting of days continues until the end of the days the medication should be completed.

The name of the medication is another very crucial part of a medical record. Whether the medication is original or generic, its name needs to appear on the medication order. A drug name is said to be a brand name when it is actually protected by some patent, usually one that the company originating with the drug holds. Such a company will have carried out the necessary tests and received approval from the FDA before making the drug available for use by the public.

A generic drug is one that is just like the original but is manufactured following the procedures used by the makers of the original drug, but after the expiration of the original company's patent rights. Generic drugs may go under different names but they are essentially bioequivalent to the corresponding branded drug. In effect, the generic drug is the same as the branded drug in terms of dose and strength as well as the medication's administration route. A good example is the drug, ciprofloxacin, which is the generic drug bioequivalent to the brand of antibiotic known as CIPRO.

Nurses and all other medical staff dispensing or administering medication ought to keep in mind that a drug is the actually brand when its name is given in capitals, and it is generic if its name is given in small letters. Often generics are even written in varying typeface. In case the name of the drug is illegible, the medical staff should not proceed with administration of the medication until the doctor who wrote the medical order has made the necessary clarification.

Remember making the right calculations for dosing whereas the medication being administered is wrong is not only unhelpful but has potential to be disastrous. Take the example of two drugs whose names are very close in spelling yet their uses are nowhere close – CELEBREX and CEREBYZ. While the first one treats pain as well as inflammation, the latter is used in keep seizures under control.

Another fundamental part of the medication order is the dose. A medication dose is that amount indicated on the medication record to be administered to the patient and includes the strength of that medicine. For a medication dose to be deemed to be written as it should be, it ought to contain the value of the medication and the units that value is being measured in. 10 milligrams is a good example of a medication dose. Although writing 10 milligrams as 10mg would be correct, such abbreviations are discouraged because they can easily cause confusion, especially when handwritten.

If, for example, the doctor writes 2 units of insulin in short as 2u, but in the handwriting the 'u' looks more round, the nurse might think that what is written is 20. Certainly that would be a massive error in terms of quantity of medication, but for a nurse or other diligent personnel, they would be quick to disqualify the medical order on grounds it does not have any unit of measurement if actually the doctor meant to write 20.

In short, a medication order can only be used when it is complete. And for the order to be complete it should contain the identity of the patient; the date as the time the medication order was issued; the exact name of the particular medication; the dose to be given to the patient; the route to be used in administering the medication; the patient's parameters; signature of the issuing doctor.

The issue of mistaken values and units has not been taken lightly among the medical fraternity, and as such there are medications that cannot be abbreviated as such abbreviations have been prohibited by the Joint Commission on Accreditation of Healthcare Organizations or JCAHO. In fact the commission has given a list of abbreviations prohibited for use in health facilities, which should be adhered to by all doctors. Some health facilities have gone a step further and made it a policy for all medications to be prescribed in their full names.

There is yet another important part of the medication order and that is the medication's administration route. The various routes available for administration of medication have their respective abbreviations too, and every nurse should know them off head. In fact, every member of the medical staff in charge of administering medication needs to be aware of these abbreviations as there is good reason why a doctor chooses one over others in the treatment of a given patient. You can check out these abbreviations in the section for abbreviations in this book.

# Chapter 3: Errors Associated with Medication Dosing

The importance of proper dose calculation cannot be overstated. Not only does it ensure proper medicine management, it also ensures the safety of patients. In 2012, incidents pertaining to medication errors in England and from June 2010 to June 2011 in Wales comprised 11% of the total reported medical incidents in that period, and this is as per reports received by the National Reporting and Learning System. It is a good thing that 90% of all those reported dosing mishaps did not cause the affected patients any harm, but it is bad enough that 253 of the total cases that counted up to 141,387 ended up causing grave damage to the affected patients. The saddest part is that 50 of the reported cases led to fatalities.

### *Meaning and Implications of a Medication Error*

It is right to consider medication error as any preventable event under the control of some medical professional or even the patient, with potential to cause unsuitable use of medication or even harm to the patient. This is the general definition provided by the *National Coordinating Council for Medication Error Reporting and Prevention.*

On the overall, any part within the system of medication use is susceptible to errors of medication. Examples of when medical errors can occur include when the prescription is being written, as someone is transferring the medical information onto a computer, at the phase of drug preparation or dispensing, or even at the time of the patient taking the medication, either alone or being given by a nurse or caregiver.

It is unfortunate that the Food and Drug Administration, or FDA, keeps receiving reports of alleged medication errors on a continued basis, averaging 100,000 per year across the US. On receipt of such reports, the FDA proceeds to review them and to classify them according to their causes and the error type. One of the means by which the FDA gets such reports is the *MedWatch*, which is FDA's reporting program for information related to safety as well as adverse events. Other sources of information include manufacturers of drugs, professionals in the medical field, as well as the consumers of medications themselves.

When medical errors are significant, they could have harmful impact on the patient. Some of the serious effects of medication errors include dire need for hospitalization, birth defect on an unborn baby, disability to the patient, patient facing a situation that is life threatening, and even death of the patient.

It has been established that many of the errors associated with medication happen as a result of the inappropriate dose being used or omitted, administration of medication being delayed, or even administration of inappropriate medication. This is the position as per the National Patient Safety Agency, 2009a. What is worth noting at this juncture is that most of the medical errors associated with dosing actually emanate from incorrect calculations. This then underscores the importance of mastering the skills of dosing calculations, and of doing sufficient practice so that you can do many of the calculations mentally.

### Dosing Errors Common with Nurses

- Failure to understand medication measurement units and their differences, such as nanograms versus micrograms.

- Making use of inappropriate equipment when measuring dosages.

- Making calculation errors whose result is giving a patient a dose of medicine that is wrong.

Although at times nurses can make such errors out of stress or being distracted, many times they make the errors for lack of adequate appropriate knowledge and skills. When it comes to lessons on dosage calculations, it is not only nurses across all health sectors that need them, but also other personnel in the health environment such as anesthetists, laboratory technologists, doctors and others. For different health personnel, when they are not using math to prescribe and make medical deductions, they will be making use of mathematical information to dispense medicine, to make diagnosis, or even report research findings.

### Seriousness of Dosing Errors in the US

It has already been mentioned that dosing errors are significant globally and the issue needs to be addressed to avoid unnecessary dangers to patients' health. At this juncture, we are going to put into perspective the seriousness of dosing errors in the US. Recent research has shown that this problem of medication dosing rates third as a killer in the US, coming only after heart disease and then cancer, but the problem is not very much publicized.

According to a study by Johns Hopkins, a quarter of a million people die annually in the US from errors of a medical nature. In fact in some sectors of the medical field, it is said the figures of such fatalities is as high as 440,000, and there are some advocacy groups and individuals putting in effort to fight for stronger legislation that ensures better safety for patients.

In early 2018, CNBC.com carried a story of a man speaking of her daughter's untimely death that had occurred 2yrs earlier, after some pharmacy technician put an overdose in the girl's intravenous or IV bag. Shockingly, the dosage miscalculation had led to the technician giving Emily Jerry a dose twenty times more of the sodium chloride prescribed for her chemotherapy session. The father, Christopher Jerry, was greatly saddened by the fact that the daughter had endured several surgeries and chemotherapy and even beaten a huge abdominal tumor, only to die during her final chemo session due to a simple mathematical error, instead of celebrating her second birthday with a story of medical success.

The main reason statistics of medical errors from different researchers vary is that doctors, funeral directors, and even coroners as well as medical examiners are not often known to highlight the aspect of human error involved in a patient's death, or even errors associated with the medical system. Yet the Center for Disease Control and Prevention depends on death certificates when recording death related statistics across the country. Due to the obvious inadvertent misinformation, the research team from Johns Hopkins University School of Medicine that was led by Dr. Makary, in their report, put an appeal to the CDC to modify the manner it gathers its data.

### Evidence of Effort to Reduce Dosing Errors

Despite the worrying figures of medical dosing errors, things are looking bright as there is evidence that governments are making an effort to ensure their citizens are protected from errors associated with prescriptions and other medical services.

For example, in the US, the FDA has expanded its scope of regulation to include the manner in which manufacturers display crucial information on over-the-counter (OTC) medications. The FDA being a federal agency, it means its requirements must be met by manufacturers of medicines all over the country.

### Exact Measures taken by FDA to Minimize Medication Errors

The FDA takes its role seriously in trying to keep patients safe, and one of the measures the agency has taken is to thoroughly review the names of drugs and their packaging as well as labeling, before it can approve the drug for marketing. During this review stage, the agency also checks the design of the product with a view to identifying any information likely to lead to medication errors, and ensuring that such information is reviewed before the product can be introduced to the market.

### Specific Aspects of Drugs Reviewed by FDA

The drug aspects the FDA monitors to ensure patient safety include the names suggested by drug manufacturers for their brands. As far as the FDA is concerned, the name must not cause confusion among consumers. In this regard, the agency makes use of prescriptions in simulated form as well as models that are computerized. In carrying out this exercise, the FDA's idea is to determine how acceptable the suggested proprietary name is with regard to causing minimum medication errors. In short, the name is accepted by the FDA only if the agency is satisfied the product name is unlikely to mislead the consumer in any adverse manner.

Another aspect the FDA is keen about pertains to the labeling of the drugs. The agency calls for proper labeling so that patients are not easily confused while taking the medications. For example, the FDA proposes putting some difference in the labeling even within the same brand, to make it easy for a patient to differentiate just by looking the container for the 5mg tablets, 10mg tablets, 25mg tablets and so on. The agency also demands varying colors within a given label design for the sake of identifying medications of the same brand but of varying strengths, or alternatively putting the units for different strengths in clear bold letters as well as numbers.

Another aspect checked keenly by the FDA is the manner in which the information meant for the patient is delivered, inclusive of the manufacturer's prescribing instructions and the directions pertaining to drug preparation. All these, according to the FDA, need to be written with simplicity and to be clear enough to read.

Once the FDA has approved particular drugs for the US market, the agency embarks on monitoring the use of the drug with a view to assessing if there are any reports of medication errors associated with those specific drugs. For example, even after a drug has been approved, the FDA can still instruct the manufacturer to adjust its labeling or packaging, or even the drug's design. The agency might even demand that the manufacturer changes the drug's proprietary name. All these adjustments are proposed in a bid to alleviate errors of dosing calculations or other medical nature.

It is also not unusual to see the FDA issue some public communication pertaining to a particular drug, to alert the populace of some breach of safety standards by the manufacturer. Such communication may be in form of Drug Safety Alerts; Drug Safety Podcasts; Medication Guides; or even Drug Safety Communications.

There is good collaboration between the FDA and various stakeholders and regulators, as well as organizations dealing with the safety of patients, when it comes to establishing causes of various medical errors. These entities include ISMP, which is the Institute for Safe Medication Practices, and organizations known for setting standards like the US Pharmacopeia.  In their collaboration, the parties seek to identify appropriate interventions so that errors already discovered are not repeated, and also to explore safety issues on a wider scale with a view to pre-emptying any incidences that may lead to medication related errors.

The FDA has takes seriously the issue of ensuring the correct medication gets to the right patient at the correct dosage, and to accomplish this the agency has enacted rules that require given drugs to have barcodes. Barcodes are effective in enabling medical professionals to carry out verification of a particular drug by use of scanning equipment, which ensures the drug delivered is the correct one. The rules the agency sets up are also meant to ensure medication is administered at the correct dosage and also at the appropriate time. The systems the FDA puts in place are actually geared towards reducing incidences of errors associated with medication prevalent in hospitals and different other health settings.

It should be easy for any diligent manufacturer or medical practitioner to get the information and guidelines provided by the FDA, as the agency has ensured these are published. Even a manufacturer who is new in the market can easily get FDA's guidelines pertaining to label designs for their medication, packaging, and even selection of an appropriate name. If all stakeholders were to adhere to FDA's guidelines, errors linked to medication dosage and other related mistakes could be minimized.

To have a glimpse of FDA's guidelines, you can look at the *Safety Considerations for Product Design to Minimize Medication Errors* issued in 2016, where it is clear the agency is focused on safe usage of medication.

### FDA's Recommendations in the 2016 Guidelines

The forms that bear instructions for the use of tablets, or any other form used for dosage, must contain imprint codes that are not only distinct but legible. The purpose for such clarity is to ensure that the health providers making prescriptions and dispensing medicine are able to easily verify the exact drug within the product as well as its strength. The information needs to be clear enough even for the patient to read it.

Also any devices for dosing packaged alongside the medicine, such as oral syringes packed alongside oral medication, must be suitable for the recommended dosage or the dosage expected to be measured. For example, if the dosage provided is in milliliters, it is only reasonable that the oral syringe packed alongside the medicine is labeled in milliliters.

There have been occasions where errors in dosing have occurred because whereas the medication dosage was provided in milliliters the labeling on the oral syringe was provided in milligrams.

The packaging design of the medication ought to be such that it is unlikely for the consumer of the product to confuse its usage. This means the packaging design of oral medication should be quite different from that of medication used for external use, or topical medications. The containers should particularly look distinctly different.

Such distinction helps to minimize medical errors such as those leading to patients putting medication used for the skin in their ears or eyes or even in the nose or mouth.

It is important to note that the FDA could do its best to ensure manufacturers of medicinal products give out the right information in the right manner, but errors of dosing can only be kept at the minimum when every medical practitioner is adept at dosage calculations. That is why technicians, nurses and everyone else involved in dosage of medication at any level ought to keep polishing their skills of dosage calculations, so as to ensure they do not contribute to the unsettling number of medical errors and unwarranted fatalities.

# Chapter 4: Math in the Field of Medicine

Mathematics is about finding solutions to problems. To be good at mathematics, you need to be able to think in a logical way and to do what it takes to find a solution to a problem. There are several ways you can use to tackle math as a science, especially because math is found almost everywhere in people's lives, whether individuals are conscious of it or not.

We all use mathematics in our day to day lives, whether we are drafting a budget, calculating our time schedules or even figuring out discounts and gratuities. For you to operate effectively in your work place, it is important that you are familiar with basic principles of mathematics. This is because, whether you work in the field of medicine or as an hourly worker, you will need to apply math at some point in your daily tasks.

### *Importance of Math to the Physician*

As a physician, you need to have an understanding of how the body works for you to be able to determine what a person is suffering from and what medication they need to be put under. For example, once a complete blood count test is carried out in a lab to determine the blood cell level in the body, a physician should be in a position to interpret the results as received from the lab.

With the help of mathematics, you can interpret ratios and percentages of the different cells and establish the overall health of your patient. Unusual results will tell you what issues need to be addressed and so on. Once you have identified any ailment and also determined the appropriate medication, you now need to decide the correct treatment dosage. Luckily, this you can achieve by using the patient's weight as the standard unit of measurement, and this is largely a mathematical approach.

### *Using Math to Maintain Patients' Health*

It is true that some of the best ways that you can keep track of a patient's progress is by maintaining a good doctor-patient relationship as well as listening keenly to a patient's feedback. However, mathematics and figures have proven over time that they are great at determining the actual health condition of a patient. Some of the roles of a doctor include analyzing CAT scans and X-rays, evaluating the medical history of a patient such as their weight, height, blood cell count and their blood pressure, as well as creating graphs that indicate the occurrence of a certain epidemic or how successful certain treatments have been over time. Needless to say, all these activities use math in one way or another.

### Using Math to Determine Suitable Prescription

As a doctor, you are required to write prescriptions for your patients and this involves a lot of math such as multiplication, addition and subtraction. For example, you are required to state how many times a particular medication should be taken in a day, the exact dosage to be taken and how long that dosage should last. With such information, you are also able to order medication that will last the patient until their next visit. Remember that you should determine the right dosage to prescribe to a patient by measuring their weight.

### How Math is Helpful to Nurses

Nurses are required to have good mathematical skills because other than taking care of their patients, their work also involves calculations and estimations. For example, for you to determine the number of heart beats per minute, you should count how many heart beats can be felt in about five seconds then multiply that number by twelve since there are 60 seconds in a minute. Another area where you are required to use math is when using an IV drip. Here you need to know exactly how much IV fluid is needed and at what rate it ought to flow so that the patient receives the right dosage. Understanding measurements also enables you to measure oxygen levels found in a patient's bloodstream as well as the quantity of urine and other fluids passed.

In order for you to administer the correct amount of medicine, you need to know simple math such as fractions, addition, subtraction, algebraic equations and ratios. This is so important that nursing students have to enroll for a mathematics class as a mandatory unit in their studies.

### General Use of Math in Dosage Calculations

Medicine is administered in different dosages depending on factors such as weight and the medicine's level of effectiveness. With this being the case, you have to do some calculations in cases where the medication is not packaged in its exact dosage. For example, if you are required to administer a 600mg dosage to a patient but the tablets are only packaged in 200mg, then you need to figure out exactly how many tablets you will have to give that will be equivalent to 600mgs. In the same way, when giving an injection, one must calculate the amount of medicine in ml to be drawn up in the syringe.

### Use of Math Skills to Convert Units between Varying Systems

Traditionally, most Americans use the apothecary system or household measurements such as Fahrenheit for temperature, and pounds, inches and ounces for other specific measurements. However, while measuring medicine, we mainly use a metric system and this requires that you have good conversion skills. You should be able to convert pounds to kilograms, inches to centimeters, ounces to centimeters cubed, degrees Fahrenheit to degrees Celsius and so on.

### Using Math in Calculation of Rates of IV Drip

In some cases, IV medicine is not given using an electric pump. In such situations, there is need for you to calculate the exact amount of fluid to be administered in form of drops. Usually, a large IV fluid bag can hold 1,000 cubic centimeters of fluid. If one bag of 1,000cc is intended to last for 6 hours, then you must calculate how many drops should be administered per minute over the period of the 6 hours.

### How Math Helps in Drug Titration

Drug titration, a case where prescribed medication is prepared from two different solutions by the dispensing staff, is often done by specially trained and experienced nurses because it requires sharp and focused mathematical skills to get it right. A physician can order for drug titration depending on a patient's condition and this requires that the medication be administered in the specified amounts. This is an example of instances where proficiency in math calculations proves invaluable.

### Other Ways Competence in Math is Handy

There are other places that nurses and physicians are needed to use their mathematical skills other than in giving medication. In some cases such as when you are handling a diabetic patient, you may be required to calculate how many calories have been taken in through the day, in order to determine what kind of care your patient needs.

You are also able to calculate how much fluids in cubic centimeters have been given to a patient and how much has been wasted through either vomiting or pouring. This, in turn helps you know how much of a particular fluid needs to be dispensed all through the day. Some nurses are also specialized in calculating the ovulation dates of a patient, glycemic index, body-mass index, pregnancy due dates and other data oriented tests, all of which require skills in math.

### How Pharmacists Make Use of Math Skills

As a pharmacist, a lot of activities require calculation, and it is therefore important for you to have a strong background in both science and mathematics. Many dosages require some mathematics to formulate and so you must understand ratios, percentages and other measurements for you to put together the correct dosage. You should also know simple concepts such as adding, subtracting and multiplying so that you can give the correct number of pills to the patient under your care.

### The Role of Math in Health Related Careers in General

Mathematics plays a big role in the field of health care and so as a health care provider, you need to have some basic mathematic skills to ensure that everything runs smoothly. When you collect essential data and figures on a disease or epidemic, you should be in a position to interpret and use that information in identifying and treating the disease. Also you need to be able to put preventive measures in place.

Mastering formulas, units of measurement and all relevant healthcare tools should enable you work efficiently. The skills will also help to greatly reduce your chances of causing medical mistakes such as giving an over dose to a patient. Some medical mistakes have potential to cause tragedies, which sometimes can even attract cases of malpractice in court of law.

### Role of Math in Taking of Vital Signs

It is important for you to know how to read and interpret the units of measurement in use as you measure patients' vital signs such as a patient's pulse rate, temperature, blood pressure and breathing rate. For example, for the large lines on a blood pressure gauge, each measures 10millimeters Hg while the small lines represent 2mmHg.

When using a non-digital thermometer to measure temperature, you are expected to know that the long line represents 1° Fahrenheit while the small notches represent 0.3°. Without knowledge on such measurements, you are likely to misinterpret the results and consequently misdiagnose the patient.

### The General Role of Math in Dispensing Drugs

A lot of conversions are done when dispensing drugs and so you need to know how to convert different units of measurements without much effort. For example, when you are supposed to give a patient 2 grams of a particular medication every six hours and medication available is in form of 500 milligram pills, you should be able to calculate that 1,000 milligrams make one gram and so for you to give 2 grams of medicine, you then need 4 pills of 500 milligrams each.

### The Role of Math within the Operation Room

Anesthesiologists must use mathematics in formulating the correct solution doses for patients who are about to undergo surgical procedures, such as converting pounds into kilograms. You need to first of all measure a patient's weight so as to determine how much of a particular medication should be given and in what ratio, if the medication is in solution form. Using the correct measurements ensures that the medicine is not too strong to the point that it can cause harm to the patient's vital organs, or even cause paralyses. At the same time, it ensures that the medication is not so mild that it becomes ineffective. You should also be able to measure and give the right amount of oxygen to a patient who needs oxygen support during the operation. In procedures such as plastic or facial surgery, a physician uses math-generated monitoring models that illustrate the procedure's results.

### How Math Helps in Effective Running of Health Facilities

As a health data analyst you are responsible for collecting helpful numerical data and performing calculations that help health facilities in serving their patients. Information such as a sudden increase in booked patients and patients visiting a facility with similar or the same health conditions can point out to an outbreak of sorts or an epidemic. Certainly this would need to be addressed. In the same way, when you have data on how many patients are booked into the hospital and how long their stay often is, you are in a position to come up with an efficient scheduling plan in order to avoid issues such as double booking or crowding.

In general, all healthcare careers require the use of mathematics in order to carry out their respective roles. As an accountant, you are required to calculate the losses and profits of health facilities, and when reporting on revenue, you should tally reimbursements made by insurance companies, money given by the government, direct cash payments and all other forms of cash in order to give a comprehensive report on all the institution's assets.

Healthcare administrators, on the other hand, are responsible for overseeing finances, preparing reports for all stakeholders, as well as creating budgets. All these tasks call for great math skills.

# Chapter 5: Medication Dosing for Special Demographics

When determining dosage for children and pregnant women, great care needs to be taken as they are, in various ways, vulnerable. These categories of patients and other special demographics like women who are breastfeeding, people living with diabetes or kidney ailments, or even those with liver impairment, need to have their dosing considered in a way that is different from the average adult. Sometimes you may even come across summarized documentation made for public consumption regarding medicinal products and their characteristics, and especially how they affect the special categories of patients.

In many countries there is the Summary of Product Characteristics, abbreviated as SmPC, on which pharmaceutical manufacturers base the designing and documentation on their packaging leaflets, abbreviated as PLs. These leaflets accompany the medicinal product for the sake of providing information to the public, and more so the patients, regarding the product before use. There is a generally accepted format as well as content for these leaflets, and some clinical information is mandatory. They are, especially, expected to include information regarding dosage for the special groups of patients, and also information on how the product might affect each of them.

Such information includes dosing for pediatric patients, the elderly, patients who have some major organ impairment, those undergoing treatment for significant illnesses on a continual basis, people taking medication that can easily interact with the product, and even pregnant and lactating women.

### *Special Dosing for Children*

Dosing is very important when it comes to special demographics, and medical personnel need to have information pertaining to limits and exemptions for patients in these populations. For children, it is mandatory for manufacturers of medications to spell out how the drug should be used or avoided with children. Almost always, any medication should be used differently on children from how it is used on adults.

The response children have to medication is usually different from that of adults, and for this reason particular care is necessary when prescribing medication to young ones. Doctors, nurses and other medical personnel need to ensure pediatric patients are given the appropriate dosage of medication at all times, and those in the neonatal stage are even more sensitive.

## Why Children Respond Differently to Medication

### Aspect of Oral Absorption

Tender infants do not have similar working of the gastric and even intestinal function, and this factor counts when it comes to determining the right dosing for them. Transit time within the gastric area and within the intestines is longer in very tender infants, and the time only becomes shorter and more normalized as they reach the age of 6mths. On the other hand, as these infants become older, their intestinal function tends to hasten. These variations need to be taken into account when determining how much of specific medications to administer to the patient, as they also affect the drug's retention period in the body.

### Increase in Gastric pH

This factor pertains to the output of gastric acid in the body, and for the child, the output does not measure that of an adult. In fact, the output only approaches and often reaches the level of the adult when the child is 2yrs old.

### Additional Factors Affecting Drug Absorption in Kids

There are additional factors known to affect the rate and efficiency of drug medication in children, and these include the contents in their gastrointestinal area, state of the pediatric patient's illness, and even existing interventions of a therapeutic nature like some drug therapy of sorts.

Medication Distribution

When it comes to body water, it sometimes decreases with respect to the patient's bodyweight and age. For the neonates, they actually need to be treated with drugs that are water soluble more than adults, and the dosage in terms of milligrams per kilograms this should be higher than in the prescription for adults.

Body metabolism

Some systems in the body are different from those of adults, mostly because of the rate of development and the stage in life at which they develop. Some systems, such as the enzyme system, may be entirely absent at the time of child's birth, and if present, it is only at minimal level. This is bound to affect the way foodstuff and drugs are metabolized in a child's body.

In some cases, the pathways for metabolism are different when it comes to certain drugs. For this reason, some drugs may be deemed unsuitable for children while the same drugs do exemplary well in adults.

Another factor that impacts dosing for children is the fact that the rate of metabolism in children tends to rise impressively in children as they grown, many times surpassing that of adults. For this reason, it sometimes becomes necessary to administer certain medications in children more regularly than you would do to adults. If not an increase in the dosing frequency, dosage on the basis of a milligram per kilogram is raised.

Aspect of Excretion

It is important to note that for infants, renal function does not mature completely until they have attained the age of 6mths to 8mths. This is a factor that is taken into consideration when it comes to determining the appropriate dosage for infants.

### *Drug Administration Route & Regime*

How the dosage is administered in children is determined by the taste of the medication and how it looks, the drug formulation, and also how easy it is to administer the medication as prepared.

The administration regiment needs to be tailored to suit the child's normal routine on a daily basis, and whenever feasible, the nurse or other medical personnel should collaborate with the kid. This makes compliance to the set schedule much easier than otherwise.

For school going children, it is best to avoid making it necessary for the child to take medication at school time. There are different ways of achieving this, one of them being prescribing drugs whose release has been modified, or even drugs that have longer half lives. However, it is understandable that it could be difficult to adjust some medications where frequency of administration is concerned, but in such cases, the child could be given some medication specifically to be taken during school time, where the times of administration are set to match the school's daily routine. If this step is taken, the dose for school should be labeled distinctly different from the medication meant to be taken at home.

Different schools accommodate pupil's personal needs differently, and while in some schools the administration may request the parents or guardians to instruct the school in writing to administer particular medication to their children, others may request that the parents and guardians make time to go to school and administer the medication themselves.

It is also recommended to avoid, as far as feasible, administration routes that would cause pain to children, a good example being intramuscular or IM injections.

Although many medications meant for children are licensed as such, there are some that are fit for the pediatric patients but are not exclusively licensed for this use. Whenever the doctor finds that some medication originally meant for adults or for general use to be good for a young patient, the nurse should be keen to keep to the exact dosage as prescribed by the doctor.

In fact, there is a provision in the European legislation, Medicine Act of 1968, which allows doctors to prescribe medications differently from the way it is presented on the label, although the doctor should be able to support such use in advance, taking into account the child's safety and efficacy of the medication.

### *Manner of Writing a Prescription*

When writing a prescription for a child who is below 12yrs old, it is necessary to include the child's age on the prescription. In fact, whenever prescribing any medication for a child, it is always preferable to state the child's age. It is also very important that the strength of the medication being prescribed be indicated in the prescription, especially when it comes to capsules or other tablets.

Liquid medications are found to be suitable for children, but sometimes they also put the children at risk of tooth decay because of the sugar added to them to encourage the children to like it. So, if the treatment is being prescribed on a long-term basis, it is preferred that the medication recommended be free of sugar. This should not pose any significant problems since many children are capable of swallowing capsules and even tablets as they are in their solid state. This is another instance where the doctor is encouraged to have a discussion with the pediatric patient and the parents, so that they are on the same page when choosing the best formulation for the child.

When the prescription being used has the medication in liquid form and the dose to be administered is below 5 milliliters (mL), one should expect an oral syringe to be provided.

### *Warning to Guardians of Kids*

Parents are discouraged from adding prescribed medications to the child's food even if they think it is easier to ingest the medication that way, and the medical personnel should tell the parents as much. The reason for this precaution is that there is a chance that the medication could interact with milk or any other liquid serving as the child's food. In addition, the child may end up consuming less medication than the amount in the dosage if it does not consume all the liquid food provided.

Although there is some discretion left for the doctor in special circumstances, they should always seek to provide dosage as the guidelines in the reference manual for pediatric dosage. They should not ignore this and embark on extrapolating a child's dosage from a given adult dose. In short, you should not take children as mini adults but as patients under their own category, which is children.

There are defined age ranges considered to be suitable guidelines when it comes to dosage for children, and you can see them here below.

- Pre-term or child whose birth comes before 37wks

- Neonate or child whose age is from birth up to 1mth

- Infant or child whose age is from 1mth up to 12mths

- Child or one whose age begins at 1yr up to 12yrs

- Adolescent or one whose age begins at 12yrs up to 18yrs

Whenever children dosage is given on the medication details without mention of age, it should be assumed the information pertains to patients whose age is 12yrs and below.

### *About Dosage Calculations for Children*

There are instances where medical personnel calculate doses for children in relation to adults, but this is with respect to the child's age and weight, the surface area of the patient's body. Sometimes more than one of those factors is taken into consideration.

Where body weight is a factor, the medication dose is expressed in terms of milligrams per kilogram (mg/kg). For children who are pretty young, the dose given is often higher per kilogram than it is for adults, and this is because of the varying metabolic rates for these two age groups.

In case the doctor has reason to think the dosage might exceed what is required by prescribing amount per kilogram of body weight, there is the alternative of relying on the ideal body weight, which you get by calculating the weight with respect to the child's height as well as age. Another method sometimes used in prescribing medication for children deals with estimates of the patient's surface area, and this is because there are several aspects of a child's physiology that have some correlation with the child's surface area of the body.

When doctors choose to use a child's height as well as weight, they find reliance on a nomogram more reliable, but they can also use other modern programs to calculate dosage on the basis of a pediatric patient's BSA or body surface area. The reason dosage aided by a nomogram is often preferred is that a nomogram, which is basically a form of a diagram, bases its dosage calculation not only on the child's body weight and age, but also on the child's gender and condition of the patient's renal function.

### Adverse Reactions to Medication

Adverse reactions to medication can differ in children in comparison to the reaction in adults. However, the important thing is for doctors, pharmacists and other medical personnel to report to the relevant authorities any suspected reactions deemed to be adverse to patients. Whether it is an adult or a child patient who has experienced advance reactions after consuming the medication it needs to be reported so that investigations can be carried out and other potential users of the medication can be saved the danger beforehand.

### Importance of Reporting Adverse Reactions in Children

- Children may react differently to a drug from an adult

- Many times the effect of drugs is not sufficiently tested in kids.

- There are several drugs being prescribed 'off label', meaning they have not been particularly licensed to be dispensed to children.

- There may be lack of appropriate formulations in the market to enable medical practitioners to prescribe dosage that is precise to children.

- The same ailment may present differently in children as compared to adults, and the likewise the reactions may also vary.

### Minding Home Safety for Children

It is important for medical personnel to warn parents on the need to ensure medications are kept away from children's reach. All doses of a solid nature as well as oral and liquid preparations meant for external use need to be reserved in containers that are child resistant. However, such containers should be convenient for the adults or guardians to open. Also, whenever feasible, medications that remain in pharmacies and probably expire before use ought to be returned to the supplier so that the supplier can destroy them.

## Special Dosing for the Elderly

Medics have information pertaining to dosing for the elderly patients, and that information is to do, among other things, when it is necessary to adjust doses of medication, how to relate the dosage to the patient's body metabolism and also risks specific to the elderly.

Elderly people have been observed to use herbal medication even as they continue to seek pharmaceutical treatments, either using doctors' prescriptions or through over-the-counter medication purchases. In the US, a survey conducted around 2010/2011 found that adults whose age bracket is within 62 – 85 years of age tended to use some medications more regularly than others, with one prescription drug being used by a whole 87% of the over 2,000 adults comprising the sample. It was also established that a good 38% relied on over-the-counter medication drugs.

On the overall, the elderly are among the demographic that consumes medications a lot. Medicare also had opportunity to do some survey and they observed that patients under Medicare who had been discharged and had left institutions of acute hospitalization, ending up in some facility of skilled nursing, were living on a prescription of 14 different medications on average. Of that array of medications, a third of produced in those elderly people side effects with potential to exacerbate the patients' original ailments.

Patients of that age group that is relatively elderly also rely a lot on herbal medications that sometimes pass as dietary supplements. Good examples are ginseng, glucosamine, and extracts from the ginkago biloba plant. The population of elder patients using herbal medication has basically risen from a paltry 14% going by 1998 statistics to a whole 63% based on statistics of 2010. In fact, in a study that examined 3,000 adult ambulance patients aged 75yrs and above, about 75% of them were confirmed to have been using one prescription drug at the minimum, and also one dietary supplement.

The importance of such studies is to make medics aware of the need to ask questions to patients regarding their use of herbal medication in addition to inquiring about other prescription medications. There is one study in the US that revealed the lack of inquiry on the part of medical staff regarding herbal medications the patients are already using. 75% of those interviewed in that study, who had already attained the age of 18yrs of age, said they had not been asked about their use of unconventional treatments when they found themselves in hospital or in a doctor's clinic. Incidentally, patients themselves do not find it necessary to disclose the information to doctors regarding their use of herbal medications or any other treatments that are not considered conventional forms of treatment.

### Why Medics Should Inquire About Use of Herbal Medication

Medicines extracted from plants are used for treatment because they are potent in medication properties. As such, if taken alongside some pharmaceutical treatments, the patient could be overdosing. In addition, there is potential for medications from herbs to interact with other therapies prescribed by the doctor, and this can be risky to the patient. This underscores the importance of inquiring from patients if they are currently using herbal medications or undergoing any unconventional treatments. Take the example of the much liked extract from ginkgo biloba. If consumed at the same time you happen to be using warfarin, you can find yourself experiencing unwarranted bleeding. Warfarin is normally prescribed as an anticoagulant. Another herbal treatment that is known to interact with modern medicines is St. John's wort. If elderly adults take this one with inhibitors of Serotonin uptake, it can easily lead to a condition termed serotonin syndrome. In fact, a certain survey carried out on 22 herbal supplements and involved patients whose age was within the range of 60 to 99 years established that there is certainly risk of interaction between herbal supplements and other medications. Needless to say, excessive bleeding occasioned by the interaction between pharmacy medications and herbal supplements can be a threat to the patient's health and life in general, and doctors, nurses and everyone else should guard against such risks.

### How to Ascertain Quality in Prescribing for the Elderly

There are several factors contributing to the general suitability of a given drug, and also its quality on the overall. Such factors include avoiding medications that are deemed unsuitable for the old, using prescribed medications as instructed, taking note of any side effects and reporting them immediately, ensuring the patient maintains the requisite drug level during the period of treatment, avoiding drugs known for having interactions, as well as involving the concerned patients in the treatment process. There is also need to take into account the values of the individual patient when making decisions that appertain to the patient's treatment.

### The Issue of Polypharmacy

By polypharmacy is meant a person's use of several medications at a go. Medical practitioners need to be aware of the different medications a patient is taking as they embark on treating the patient. As highlighted in the cases involving use of unconventional treatments, some treatments have potential to interact and put the patient's health in jeopardy.

There is sometimes debate as to when to consider a patient a subject of polypharmacy since there is no set minimum number of medications to warrant the term, but in practice, any patient taking five medications upwards, and even up to ten, can be said to be involved in polypharmacy. One thing medical practitioners should do more of is taking into account any health supplements the patient is taking when assessing the patient for polypharmacy. Of course, over-the-counter medications should be taken into account too, as opposed to considering just the medications the doctors have prescribed.

## Why Polypharmacy is a Concern

This issue of polypharmacy becomes a concern when you consider the potential of some medications interacting, and it is even a bigger issue where the elderly are concerned. In comparison to younger people, those of advanced age have a tendency to experience more health conditions, and hence to have more prescriptions given to them. According to Medicare, 20% of its beneficiaries suffer from up to five health conditions of a chronic nature, and 50% of them actually consume five medications or even more concurrently. Within the population of elderly patients with cancer but who are still able to walk on their own, 84% of them were noted in some study to be consuming five different medications and sometimes more, whereas 43% were noted to be receiving 10 medications or even more.

There is evidence that use of a wide range of medications increases the risk of drug related events of an adverse nature, commonly referred to as ADE. The issue of adverse drug event is relevant whether the patients concerned are old or young, and has many times necessitated patient admission. It has also been noted that polypharmacy can result in reduced physical capacity as well as minimized cognitive capacity. That is one important reason why medical practitioners should seek to get information regarding patients' use of other medications prior to making their medication orders.

## Why the Elderly are more adversely impacted by Polypharmacy

One of the reasons elderly individuals are more likely to be adversely affected by polypharmacy is that their metabolic rate is always changing, and the rate of drug clearances keeps dropping as people age. These factors are compounded as the range of medications the individual is taking becomes wider. Polypharmacy is also known to increase the possibility of drugs interacting amongst themselves. They may also cause medical practitioners to prescribe additional medications that would not have been necessary were it not for the interactions of the other drugs.

Among the studies done regarding the elderly and dosing, it was noted in one that polypharmacy often increased the risk of hip fractures in patients. As for polypharmacy causing a medical practitioner to prescribe additional medications, it is because the interaction of the numerous medications makes the patient appear to be experiencing an entirely new medical condition.

Even without interactions, there is still the potential for the elderly patients to forget when and how to take their numerous medications, a fact that is compounded by many of the patients' impairment is seeing and cognition. It was found in one study conducted in 2017 that some complications emanating from medication use have to do with the patients' non-adherence to the regimen as provided by the doctor.

As for medical practitioners, they need to try and always find a balance between under prescribing medications to patients and over prescribing. Of course, it is understandable that there are times when an elderly patient has a wide range of ailments that complicate the particular patient's overall health condition, and the doctor has a big task deciding what guidelines specific to individual illnesses to adhere to. It would not be surprising, for example, to have an elderly patient diagnosed in the same period with chronic obstructive pulmonary disease and hypertension, diabetes type 2, as well as ostereoarthritis and osteoporosis. To provide proper treatment to such a patient while following the professional guidelines provided, the medical practitioner would have to prescribe for such a patient 12 different medications.

Nevertheless, after considering the dangers that come with polypharmacy, doctors are given discretion to choose the medications to discontinue and which ones to substitute. All in all, the dosing medical personnel give should match the health condition of the patient as well as the goals of health care set.

### Dosing Considerations Specific to the Elderly

There is need to re-evaluate the suitability for different medications in the late years of a patient's life. In fact, there is a model now that guides medical practitioners on how to determine the appropriateness of certain medications with respect to the patient's age. This guide takes into account the balance of the patient's life expectancy as well as the care anticipated when considering a review of the patient's medication.

For example, you may have a patient who has a balance of life expectancy that can be said almost with certainty to be short, and the intention for providing additional medication is palliative. In such a case, it would not make much sense to recommend medication like some prophylactic, whose impact can only be realized many years down the line. Such considerations are now being taken to be realistic, especially in the health management of people whose dementia is at an advanced stage. Even medications such as antibiotics to treat ailments such as pneumonia cannot be guaranteed to increase the patient's comfort. In fact, such treatment cannot be guaranteed to increase the patient's life quality if the objective is to provide palliative care to the patient.

## How to Tailor Adult Prescription to Suit the Elderly

When it comes to the elderly, it is best to try and optimize medication therapy as part of their overall care. The prescribing method is often complex, as it has different sides to it. For one, the medical practitioner needs to decide if the drug is indicated, and ultimately select the drug that is safest for such an elderly person. It is best to determine the dose well and to create a schedule suitable for the physiology of the patient. It is also recommended that you monitor not only the effectiveness of the prescribed medication, but also any toxicity associated with it. You also need to educate the patient regarding any anticipated side effects. It is important to instruct the patient to report or consult on any indications noticed.

It is a fact some ADEs, or Avoidable Adverse Events, can be very serious and sometimes fatal, and this is a fact that needs to be borne in mind every time you are evaluating an elderly patient with a view to writing a prescription. Any symptom being noticed in the patient that did not exist before should be associated with the new treatment until there is sufficient proof the symptom has nothing to do with the prescribed drug.

Some challenges doctors face when prescribing are unique to elderly patients. For starters, it is not usual for the elderly to be involved in pre-marketing trials of new drugs, and so the doses given to such patients are just approximations that may not necessarily be the right doses. With that in mind, it is important to be cautious when ordering medications for elderly patients. This is especially important considering there are some changes that the elderly go through that affect absorption of drugs, their distribution, their body metabolism and excretion, processes that can be summed up as pharmacokinetics. Even pharmacodynamics, or the drug effects of a physiological nature, is also an issue.

Extra care should also be taken when determining the level of dosage as you prescribe for elderly patients, keeping in mind the possibility of distribution volume increasing due to increased proportion of fat gauged against the adult's skeletal muscle; a normal development as people advance in age. Another crucial factor to consider is the decline in the speed at which drug gets cleared from the body. The reality is that as people age their renal function also becomes less efficient, and even though the elderly person may not suffer any renal ailment, the overall renal function is still not at optimal. The decline in this function is the one that reduces the rate at which drug is cleared from the body and this should be taken into account when ordering the frequency at which prescribed medication is to be administered.

It is worth noting that when the body retains huge reservoirs of medications and then the process of drug clearance from the body is elongated, the concentration of the drug in the plasma of the blood is bound to rise, and this is precisely the case with elderly people taking medications.

Take the example of the drug, diazem. If the distribution volume for this drug increases and in the meantime the same person takes lithium whose rate of clearance remains low, as is expected in elderly people, the very same medication dose for the two drugs is likely to cause higher concentrations in the plasma where elderly people are concerned. Sometimes it is not even the drug retention or clearance that may affect the health of an elderly patient. It is simple sensitivity. As some people age, they develop sensitivity to some drugs, and benzodiazepines are a good example. Opiods, too, are in this category of medications that people are likely to become sensitive to as they advance in age.

The hepatic function is another of the body functions that declines as people age. Some of the changes affecting this function and are linked to aging include changes in the efficiency in medication metabolism. This becomes even more significant in situations where polypharmacy is an issue. As the hepatic function becomes more inefficient, the elderly patient could develop sensitivity to some of the medications prescribed. In short, ADRs, or Adverse Drug Reactions, are negative effects medics should anticipate as they embark on issuing prescriptions to elderly patients.

### *Dosing Unsuitable for the Elderly*

The elderly are generally recognized as a vulnerable demographic, and it is for this reason that countries like Canada and the US have embarked on assessing the quality maintained in prescribing medications to the members of this age group. There is even criteria termed 'Beers criteria' that regulates how dosing should be done with regards to elderly persons.

In general, what these guidelines and others under different indices seek to achieve is best quality of healthcare for elderly persons, as effort is made to ensure their bodies are not overburdened with medications with potential to harm them in due course. Special attention is given to medications with sedative effect and even anticholinergics, as well as everyday dosing and the collection of medications involved. Medications such as those cited have been found to cause impairment of sorts to the elderly, especially where mobility and cognition is concerned. For instance, the drug, Zolpidem, has in the past been implicated in 21% of cases of patients over 65yrs of age reporting at the emergency department, and this is following adverse effects experienced by the patients after having prescribed the drug dosage for psychiatric related illnesses.

Although the large number of medications prescribed has not been linked directly to cognitive or suchlike impairment, in the long run elderly people under such medications somehow become prone to falls as they move around within the health care facilities or wherever else they dwell. When it comes to medications that are anticholinergic, meaning medications such as clidinium, atropen and the like, they are linked to a myriad of side effects when used in treatment, and the elderly are particularly affected.

That notwithstanding, it was established in a study that took place from 2005 to 2009 that this category of medications are still very much in use, with dementia patients of over 65yrs old receiving prescriptions of medications with great level of anticholinergic activity. Sadly, these medications are often the cause of memory impairment for these elderly individuals, vision blurriness and nausea, confusion and hallucinations, and other side effects like urinary retention, constipation and dry mouth, and even abnormal sweating as well as tachycardia. In fact, anticholinergic medications can exacerbate acute glaucoma.

The import of this is that medical practitioners should go beyond standard dosing for adults, and take into account the special needs of vulnerable categories of patients, such as the elderly. In one study involving almost 7,000 patients, both men and women aged 65yrs and above, the individuals taking anticholinergics were found to be at higher risk of declining in their cognitive abilities and to suffer dementia. What was noted is that the risk earlier identified fell when the anticholinergics were discontinued.

In a different study involving close to 3,500 subjects of both gender aged 65yrs and above, their risk of dementia as well as Alzheimers disease heightened as dosages of anticholinergics were increased. This was more so with the prescribing of antihistamins of first generation and also tricyclic anti-depressants, as well as bladder anti-muscarinics.

### The Importance of Beers Criteria

The criteria referred to as Beers Criteria was founded by some expert panel of consensus back in 1991, and the panel's target was residents of nursing homes. They felt those were the main patients experiencing poor prescribing methods and the situation needed to be rectified.

This panel came up with a list comprising medications thought to be unsuitable for the elderly demographic, and they based their decision on how ineffective a particular drug was and also the level of risk the drug posed to the patient. The findings of the panel, and hence the criteria, happens to have support from the 'American Geriatrics Society, which advices clinicians to ensure they take into account several factors while prescribing medications for elderly patients. In addition to doing smart math calculations, the society also urges medical practitioners to exercise common sense as well as good clinical judgment when dealing with this rather vulnerable category of patients. The society underscores the need to appreciate each individual's uniqueness, and provide dosage prescriptions accordingly as far as is feasible.

### *Ways of Improving Practices in Prescribing*

Some ways you can follow to improve efficiency in prescribing medication are explained here below.

For starters, it is important do record any indications noted from a drug therapy being used for the first time by the patient, or even from a drug therapy that is newly introduced in the health sector.

It is also important to provide patients with helpful information regarding the benefits of certain medications as well as the risks linked to such treatments. Another point to be noted is the need to keep a well updated list of medications a particular patient is using, and at the same time record the response the patient is having to the treatment.

Medical practitioners also need to keep reviewing the medication treatment prescribed to a patient from time to time, and such reviews need to be an ongoing process.

The various research studies that have been done regarding medication dosage to elderly patients have triggered the urgency to point out medications that are unsuitable for elderly patients, and particularly the ones that ought to be avoided as much as possible. There is also highlight on the medications that can be prescribed but have the patient's closely monitored after the medication process has begun.

### *Why Under-Dosing is also an Issue*

Although when people discuss improper dosing they often think of over-dosing, there are cases where under-dosing of medication is also a problem, even for patients of advanced age. It is not enough to prescribe just a few tablets to an elderly patient in a bid to avoid over-prescribing, as that in itself might not constitute improvement of the patient's overall health.

Owing to the emphasis put on avoiding over-prescribing, the error has now fallen on the side of under-prescribing, which is also not good for the patients' health. A certain study showed that in two institutions for the elderly half of the patients had not received the medication doses that had been prescribed to them by medical experts, yet when it came to over-prescribing of unwarranted medications only 3° of the elderly patient, who numbered close to 400, were affected by prescription of unsuitable medication. Still, there is a different study that showed there is prevalence of both over and under prescribing in institutions for the elderly.

In fact, such shortcomings have even been noted by the US Department of Veterans Affairs that noted prescribing of unsuitable medications to veterans at the outpatient department. Among the near-200 patients used as sample, whose age was 75yrs on average, 65% of them were noted to have been prescribed medications inappropriate to them as elderly patients, while underuse of medication was noted in 64% of the sample cases. In that study, there were still elderly patients who were victims of under-utilization of medications as well as overuse of medications. These ones comprised 42% of the sample patients.

### Medication Affordability as an Issue

There are times doctors write prescriptions but their orders are not effected, meaning the patients end up not taking the ordered medications. Other times, the prescriptions are honored and the patients receive the medications, but failure sets I when the patient does not take the medication as required.

Often when patients do not use the prescriptions given to acquire medication, it is because they cannot afford to pay for the medications. This is a weakness common in countries where health insurance for the elderly is inadequate, inefficient or simply lacking.

An incentive that can help out is one of improved insurance that covers medication, and that can ensure elderly patients take home appropriate medications as they leave hospitalization to proceed to nursing homes or other places of residence. Two groups of patients were studied, one comprising patients under Medicare and another patients with no health insurance covering medications. Within the group without proper insurance cover, only 4.1% of them actually used statin, whereas a significant 27% of those under Medicare used the drug. Even in cases where the drugs were not exactly expensive, such as nitrates or even beta blockers, there was still a significant difference between the patients under reliable health insurance than those without such cover.

It was sad to note also that where patients with disabilities were concerned, even when they were under Medicare, a significant 30% of them still did not receive medical therapies as required owing to matters of cost, and it was worse when the patient had multiple handicaps.

### How to Prescribe for Expectant Patients

Writing prescriptions for women who are pregnant can prove challenging to medical practitioners who may have inadequate information relating to safety of some drugs, and it can also be a challenge when there is a risk of overestimating the risk certain medications pose. Sometimes both the patient and the doctor are in the same position of ignorance, and the doctor may be particularly cautious not to do anything that could lead to legal suit. Such situations underline the need to understand the issues that are worth considering at the time of prescribing medications to an expecting mother, and also the need to be aware of medications that are considered safe for this category of patients.

### Medical Factors Unique to Pregnant Women

It is important to take into account that between the mother and the environment of the fetus exists no barrier of a physiological nature. As such, any medication related things that you do to the mother can easily affect the fetus.

Also, how a given medication affects the fetus may be determined by the stage of gestation the mother is in. It is also important to note that for the unborn baby to remain safe despite medications prescribed to the mother, the medical practitioner needs to go beyond the stipulations of the FDA, and make use of other helpful information in practice or learnt from experience. In short, the guidelines provided by the FDA regarding medication to a pregnant mother are in themselves insufficient to protect mother and child.

It is important to be alive to the fact that both the patients and their medical providers have their own presumptions regarding the pregnancy situation and what needs to be done or omitted in relation to medications. However, the medical practitioner must be guided, as always, by the fundamental principle of doing no harm; what they term in the medical circles, Primum non nocere. This principle that is applicable all over the world is a regular reminder to medical practitioners to always think of any possibility of harm that might befall the patient if the professional took a given form of action. Although this is a principle at the heart of every medical practitioner, its weight is even more felt when the patient under consideration is one who is pregnant.

### The Choice to Make: Baby or Mother?

Whenever a medical practitioner is attending to a patient who is pregnant, there is the nagging thought of the need to save both the mother and the unborn baby, but sometimes the professional in-charge has to make a delicate decision that demands prioritization of mother and child. In such cases, what makes it tough for the doctor is the fact that the best medication for the mother's health condition may be unsuitable for the health of the unborn baby. The doctor is faced with the question of whether to order the best medication for the adult at the expense of the unborn baby, or to rely on the mother's sentiments and cultural leanings regarding such matters.

Even the pregnant woman, in such circumstances, can be conflicted. On one hand she may understand the need to take the prescribed medications as per the doctor's orders, and on the other hand may be the motherly instincts to protect the child from any potential harm from the medication drugs. However, situations are not always as negative as the conflicting thoughts may reflect, as in many instances any treatment suitable for the mother ends up having positive impact on the baby. What becomes particularly a challenge is not whether or not to treat the pregnant mother, but identifying medications that are safe for both mother and child while avoiding overestimating medication risks.

Whatever the case, there is one fact that cannot be ignored, and that is the importance of pharmacotherapy to patients, whether they are pregnant or not.

### Factors to Consider in Prescribing for Expectant Mothers

There are some factors worth considering when you are involved in prescribing medications for expectant mothers. One of them has already been mentioned, and that is the absence of a barrier between the mother's environment and the unborn baby's environment.

### Ease of Drug to Pass through the Fetus' Placenta

To understand this, visualize the fetus' placenta as having a membrane that is semi-permeable, and which, in a selective manner, permits certain substances to permeate through from the mother's environment and to reach the blood flowing into the fetus. That same membrane is also responsible for keeping out certain substances from reaching the fetus through the blood.

Unfortunately, when it comes to medications consumed by the expectant mother, the fetus' membrane has no capacity to keep out their effects. So, inevitably, the fetus is bound to be exposed to those medications even if it is to a small degree. On the overall, medications whose molecular weight is low, those described as being lipophilic, and some others, can easily pass through the placenta to reach the fetus. Some other medications cannot pass through the placenta with such ease, and great examples of such medications are insulin as well as Heparin.

### Mother's Gestational Stage

Although as mentioned above there are some substances that do not penetrate the embryo to reach the fetus, there are those that have capacity to go through and have a negative long lasting effect on the unborn baby. Good examples are teratogens, which can be in form of disease causing microbes like those that cause herpes, and even substances like mercury and potassium iodide.

It should be noted the potential negative effect meant here on the embryo could either be of a physical nature or functional. It is particularly important that mothers be safe from teratogens during their first trimester, because they could cause malformations of a structural nature in the fetus. Nevertheless, even as doctors and other medical staff ensure a pregnant mother is protected from exposure to teratogens in the first trimester, they should be diligent too during the rest of the mother's pregnancy, as the fetus is still vulnerable to other dangers.

The health of the fetus can still be negatively impacted after the first trimester, for instance, if the mother is exposed to enzyme inhibitors that convert angiotensin. During the first trimester, if the fetus came into contact with such substances they would have a tiny increase in risk of heart defect at birth, but if the same substances come into contact with the fetus in the second up to the last trimester, they could cause defects in some particular organs, or badly affect the development of the fetus in its neurologic or even behavioral aspects.

Some of the health problems that have been cited as affecting fetuses even after the first trimester due to the mother's condition include fetal oligohydramnios, which in simple terms means the fetus might fall short of the amniotic fluid. Others are neonatal anuria, which is the inability of the infant's kidneys to release urine; pulmonary hypoplasia or under-development of organs; growth inhibition within the uterus; and even death of the fetus.

### *Physiological Effects of Medications during Pregnancy*

During pregnancy, mothers are generally known to have a higher level of plasma, and the rate of glomerular filtration is increased. However, there are chances of an expectant mother developing hypoalbuminemia, meaning the level of albumin within the blood might drop to an abnormal level, yet this substance is vital in the maintenance of normal plasma levels. There is also the aspect of the mother failing to benefit from medications owing to the low plasma levels. In addition to the decreased bioavailability of important medications to the mother, the mother may also have a problem absorbing oral agents because gastric motility may have been slowed down.

Certainly not all of the mother's physiological changes warrant alterations of drug prescriptions at all times during pregnancy, but medical practitioners can make a point of identifying and ordering a suitable agent. Take into consideration a situation where the pregnant mother is expected to take several medication doses in a day. Any potential effect the particular drugs have higher chances of affecting the fetus than if the mother was having a once per day dose. This is because the drug would take faster to clear from the body than when the drug concentration in the body is higher.

This means the doctors have a role to consider a pregnant woman a special case even if the illness being treated is ordinary. They are expected to be careful with such a woman's prescription, not only in the choice of drug but also in the dosage. The nurse in charge is also expected to understand why an adult suffering a particular illness is given medication dosage that is different from what is usual, and not be tempted to instigate a change. Considering the changes that go on during pregnancy that can affect the unborn baby, it is important that doctors resist the urge to prescribe medications for pregnant mothers for ailments that can heal without medication. At the same time, they need to advice women to desist from relying on over-the-counter medications during pregnancy just because they are experiencing some disease symptom.

The culture of over-reliance on medication is sometimes risky, not only to the pregnant mother but also to the fetus, but with some information such as the one provided in this book this behavior can change. A significant number of the medications women consume during pregnancy are to do with ailments of the upper-respiratory system in form of infections, and also headaches and distress of a psychological nature. It is important that medical practitioners teach their patients that the effect of many remedies provided for colds is quite limited, and that antibiotic medication as treatment for colds as well as viral bronchitis is unsuitable. Professionals also ought to insist on lifestyle changes for pregnant mothers, coupled with ample relaxation. It is also helpful for medics to educate their patients in this demographic on methods they can use to get rid of headache without relying on medication.

A good example of such methods is biofeedback, especially when it comes to headache that is chronic. Even for some low level depression, which sometimes affects women in their pregnancy, can be treated without use of prescription or other medications. One way of addressing mild depression or even depression that has risen to moderate levels is to get psychotherapy treatment. That ensures the mother resumes her normal happy relaxed self without consuming medicinal substances with potential to harm the fetus. In short, doctors should feel confident to give pregnant mothers the option of getting treatment that is non-pharmacologic when it comes to some specific symptoms.

### *How Patient's Values Affect Treatment*

Much as physicians are well informed and may have their hearts in the right place, sometimes their position conflicts with that of their patients, and this is not any different in cases where the patients happen to be pregnant. Sometimes they are faced with cases of patients not willing to consume medication owing to their beliefs, and this can be a problem if the doctor thinks medicinal treatment is necessary at that time for the mother or baby. It then becomes the challenge for the doctor to find ways of getting the patient to accept some level of meaningful treatment.

This is one scenario that brings to the fore the additional skills needed by doctors and other medical staff, over and above the skills to prescribe and dispense medication.

Pregnant patients present at the hospital and their attitude and behavior often reflect the experiences they have had with family members or even friends, and these attitudes can become hindrances when it comes to providing the necessary medications during pregnancy. Sometimes it is not just personal experiences that play a role in making the doctor's role of prescribing medication tough, but it is also misinformation through electronic and print media.

Since it is not possible for doctors to alter any of the patients' experiences, the most reasonable thing is to question them about their fears, and issues that they may be anxious about regarding medication in general and any possible prescriptions they may be given. Incidentally, this is not a one-way street. Doctors, too, have their fears to address. It helps to admit to themselves when they are being too cautious about medication for pregnant mothers, and work towards objectivity. A doctor may be prejudiced against prescribing certain medication or more than one medication to pregnant patients, with the fear emanating from a bad experience in the past.

The doctor may have prescribed certain medication to be taken in a given frequency, and probably the pregnancy did not end well. That may have triggered the discomfort in prescribing medications for pregnant mothers, making them hold the position pregnant mothers should steer away from medication no matter the discomfort. For doctors to be objective in prescribing medication for their pregnant patients, their scientific knowledge is not sufficient. They also need to address their personal biases, prejudices and general tendencies, and that helps in building a good foundation from which to stand as they make decisions regarding prescribing for pregnant patients.

### *Prescribing Considerations When the Mother Has Health Issues*

Sometimes the patient at the doctor's clinic is not only pregnant but also ill, with conditions such as asthma, cardiac arrhythmia or even suffering migraine headache. Some of these health conditions can affect the pregnancy, while in some instances the health conditions develop owing to the pregnancy. Before prescribing any medications, it is crucial that the doctor establishes clearly what issue is dependent on the other, because if this is not clearly known, any prescription provided may be useless. In some cases the treatment might even make the health of the patient worse.

It is not a myth that pregnancies have a way of affecting women's health conditions in various ways. For example, for a woman who already had conditions such as asthma, cardiac arrhythmia or even migraine headache, pregnancy can easily make it worse, and if not medically addressed can put the lives of mother and child at serious risk. However, for health conditions such as graves and even hypertension, these become less serious as the pregnancy grows, and often doctors are confident enough about the reduced risk that they slowly wean the patient off medication. Once the doctor understands the impact a pregnancy has on the patient's health, it becomes easy to address the problem without putting the patient's health and that of the unborn child at risk. In short, it helps for the doctor to make what would be considered an informed decision regarding the health of a pregnant patient.

To help the doctor to determine if or not to write a prescription for the patient, it is best to consider the level of risk, if any, the illness poses in case it does not get treated. Many ailments can affect how the fetus develops, and the impact would be negative. There is a good example in diabetes, where failure to control the glycemic level is associated with malformations of a congenital nature. Sometimes the patient can even face spontaneous abortion or the fetus may just die. Medical conditions that are chronic and keep exacerbating periodically put the fetus in great danger whenever there is a flare up. Good examples of such health conditions include asthma and even epilepsy.

As such, whenever there is a health condition of a chronic nature in the picture, it is important that the pregnant patient continue to receive therapy on a regular basis. It also helps, whenever feasible, for a patient with a chronic health condition to have some pre-conception counseling, in order that some appropriate drug can be made available well before pregnancy. Such medication would have sufficient data to underline its safety during pregnancy. This is a great way of keeping away any health problems that would otherwise affect mother or her embryo when the disease exacerbates.

For health conditions emerging for the first time during a woman's pregnancy, the cautionary principle remains, where the doctor must answer the question as to whether the pharmacotherapy risk is or serious than that of the untreated ailment. This is the fundamental answer that helps make the most suitable choice where the issue of prescribing or not to prescribe is concerned. As long as the doctor, in all the abundance of scientific knowledge, can find the risk of prescribing reasonably lower than that of failing to prescribe, the justifiable step would be to prescribe the helpful medication despite its possible side effects.

### *How to Select Medication for Pregnant Patients*

How safe the fetus will remain during a woman's pregnancy is dependent on the overall health of the mother. You therefore need to contemplate medication during this sensitive period as being justified or not depending on your assessment of safety. It is for this reason that certain medications are recommended for pregnant mothers in the treatment of certain health conditions while others are not. It is important to note that certain medications not outright recommended for use during pregnancy are acceptable as substitutes for the best choice in case that best choice is not within reach.

Some of these health conditions can affect the pregnancy, while in some instances the health conditions develop owing to the pregnancy. Before prescribing any medications, it is crucial that the doctor establishes clearly what issue is dependent on the other, because if this is not clearly known, any prescription provided may be useless. In some cases the treatment might even make the health of the patient worse.

It is not a myth that pregnancies have a way of affecting women's health conditions in various ways. For example, for a woman who already had conditions such as asthma, cardiac arrhythmia or even migraine headache, pregnancy can easily make it worse, and if not medically addressed can put the lives of mother and child at serious risk. However, for health conditions such as graves and even hypertension, these become less serious as the pregnancy grows, and often doctors are confident enough about the reduced risk that they slowly wean the patient off medication. Once the doctor understands the impact a pregnancy has on the patient's health, it becomes easy to address the problem without putting the patient's health and that of the unborn child at risk. In short, it helps for the doctor to make what would be considered an informed decision regarding the health of a pregnant patient.

To help the doctor to determine if or not to write a prescription for the patient, it is best to consider the level of risk, if any, the illness poses in case it does not get treated. Many ailments can affect how the fetus develops, and the impact would be negative. There is a good example in diabetes, where failure to control the glycemic level is associated with malformations of a congenital nature. Sometimes the patient can even face spontaneous abortion or the fetus may just die. Medical conditions that are chronic and keep exacerbating periodically put the fetus in great danger whenever there is a flare up. Good examples of such health conditions include asthma and even epilepsy.

As such, whenever there is a health condition of a chronic nature in the picture, it is important that the pregnant patient continue to receive therapy on a regular basis. It also helps, whenever feasible, for a patient with a chronic health condition to have some pre-conception counseling, in order that some appropriate drug can be made available well before pregnancy. Such medication would have sufficient data to underline its safety during pregnancy. This is a great way of keeping away any health problems that would otherwise affect mother or her embryo when the disease exacerbates.

For health conditions emerging for the first time during a woman's pregnancy, the cautionary principle remains, where the doctor must answer the question as to whether the pharmacotherapy risk is or serious than that of the untreated ailment. This is the fundamental answer that helps make the most suitable choice where the issue of prescribing or not to prescribe is concerned. As long as the doctor, in all the abundance of scientific knowledge, can find the risk of prescribing reasonably lower than that of failing to prescribe, the justifiable step would be to prescribe the helpful medication despite its possible side effects.

### *How to Select Medication for Pregnant Patients*

How safe the fetus will remain during a woman's pregnancy is dependent on the overall health of the mother. You therefore need to contemplate medication during this sensitive period as being justified or not depending on your assessment of safety. It is for this reason that certain medications are recommended for pregnant mothers in the treatment of certain health conditions while others are not. It is important to note that certain medications not outright recommended for use during pregnancy are acceptable as substitutes for the best choice in case that best choice is not within reach.

# Chapter 6: Prescribing At the Time of Emergency

Our preparedness in the public health sector is tested best when disaster strikes. When a disaster, whether man-made or natural, occurs the long-term and short-term consequences can be devastating. The health sector has drawn important lessons from emergencies such as the Hurricane Katrina of 2005, September 11 terrorist attack in 2001 and H1N1 pandemic that occurred in 2010-2011 and now there is heightened preparedness from the local levels all the way to the national levels. The measures that have been put in place by the health sector in conjunction with all the relevant stake holders ensure that in case of a disaster, every affected individual can receive the right physical care and treatment.

When major disaster or emergencies occur, it is inevitable that the affected individuals will be affected mentally too. This is why the health sector does not only focus on strategies to provide physical care for affected individuals but also factors in the need to focus on behavioral and mental health of this individuals. Unlike physical injury that can be diagnosed and treated almost immediately, behavioral and mental problems may manifest much later which makes it hard to diagnose or address. The affected persons should therefore be monitored and counseled even way after the emergency.

However, many individuals are not able to access these mental health facilities after the emergencies due to structural barriers. A study conducted on the Hurricane Katrina victims who were seeking mental health services indicated that over two thirds of the persons had either reduced their treatment or terminated it and about half of these people sited structural barriers as the reason. In some cases also, the mental health services are offered for only a short period of time after which the initiative is dissolved which means that the affected patients have nowhere to seek help after that.

Caring for mental health patients involves providing therapeutic interventions and prescribing drugs such as psychotropic. There are tight regulations around accessing psychotropic and many other necessary drugs and only a few prescribers are legally authorized to access them. This poses a challenge for mental health service providers especially during an emergency.

### *Authority to Prescribe in Non- emergency Situations*

In the US, the body responsible for determining if a certain medication should be prescribed by authorized healthcare providers is the Federal Food and Drug Administration. For a drug to be classified as one that needs to be sold by a legally authorized prescriber, there are several factors that are considered such as toxicity levels of the drug, how adverse the side effects can be and whether the dosage should be advised by an expert. Drugs that are labeled as "controlled substances" can be potentially abused and can create physical or psychological dependence. Examples of these drugs are amphetamine which is used to manage ADHD and benzodiazepines which is used to manage anxiety among others used to treat mental health problems.

In the United States about 12% of prescriptions are labeled as controlled substances. These drugs are regulated heavily both at the state and federal levels. Drugs that are regulated under the federal law are classified into 5 schedules. Drugs that are grouped into schedule one should not to be prescribe at all for any health purpose. Drugs like Heroin fall under schedule one. They have no approved medical use and have great potential of being abused. Drugs that fall under schedule 2 to 5 can be issued but only with prescriptions. Schedule 2 drugs have a restricted usage and a high chance of abuse. On the other hand, drugs that fall under schedule 3, 4 and 5 have a reduced chance of being abused and have widely accepted uses. Drugs that are not classified in the 5 schedules are said to be non-controlled and make up for about 90% of prescription drugs.

Content regulation can also be done by federal governments on controlled substances prescriptions. The federal government requires that information such as the name of drug, issue date and directions on how to use should be included on the bottles or tablets in all prescriptions. The state government can add their requirements as well such as requiring that all prescription bear the address and name of the patient.

Through the state government, the professional law licensure is responsible for ensuring that individuals comply with the minimum requirements before they can proceed to practice in their professions. The professional licensure also creates mechanisms for the state to oversee providers.

As a health care giver you can start providing care and services to patients once you have attained a license to practice. The services provided must however fall within your scope of practice which is defined by state's licensing regulations. Practicing without a license or exceeding your scope of services permitted by your licensure can attract heavy penalties and in some cases you can face civil liability, disciplinary action or criminal sanctions. For mental health care providers such as physicians, PAs and advanced practice nurses professional licensure also includes the permit to prescribe drugs. Professional licensure is state specific and so the authority given to mental health care givers varies from state to state.

In most cases, physician assistants and advanced practice nurses are best placed to prescribe psychotropic medication to patients with mental health conditions. This is because most physicians and specially trained providers in behavioral and mental health do not take up that role. Many believe that this is partly because there are few and unevenly distributed psychiatrists in the states and also many communities depend on non-specialist providers when it comes to mental health care.

### Prescribing Authority of a Physician across States

A physician is allowed to prescribe medication in every state but for APNs and PAs, there is a limit to the type of medication they are allowed to prescribe and what circumstances they are allowed to issue prescriptions. Physician assistants are trained to only practice under a physician's supervision and within certain limits. Different states have different regulations in regard to what a PA can do and not do. For example, in West Virginia, a PA is allowed to prescribe schedule 3 through to 5 drugs as well as non-controlled drugs but they must have been in practice for about two years or more. In Missouri however a PA is allowed to prescribe schedule 3 to 5 drugs as well as non-controlled drugs but he or she should only give a 5 day prescription for schedule 3 drugs which he cannot refill thereafter.

Advanced practice nurses are authorized to provide several healthcare services such as nursing care which sometimes is done in collaboration with a physician. Their authority to prescribe medication is often dependent on the agreement made between them and the physician. However different states have different laws. In Maryland, APNs are allowed to prescribe schedule 2 to 5 drugs while in Florida it is illegal for APNs to prescribe the controlled substance drugs. In some states such as Florida, it is challenging for an APN to give the desired mental health care due to such restrictions.

Prescriptions such as psychotropic are not easily accessible and therefore providing the right care to mental illness patients becomes difficult. Worse still physicians and other specialized care givers cannot prescribe medication which makes access to these prescriptions even more difficult. Some argue that physicians have the training and background that should give them prescribing authority while others believe that physician should not be trusted with prescribing such highly dangerous medication with the risk of abuse and serious side effects because they are not trained enough for such responsibility. As it stands today, only New Mexico and Louisiana have given physicians and psychologists the authority to prescribe drugs.

### Prescribing Authority of Health Care Givers in an Emergency

There are two groups of people who need quick access to prescribing care givers or health care givers in general. These are people who had a pre-existing condition which needed prescription even before an emergency and those that need prescription to address a new condition that has been caused by the emergency. People who live with conditions such as bipolar disorder and schizophrenia need a constant supply of medication and in the event that this supply runs out, their conditions can become worse. Some people are affected greatly by emergencies and they can end up with stress related disorders such as depression, anxiety and PTSD and so they need access to prescriptions that can help in managing these conditions especially in the first few months after an emergency.

In the face of an emergency, licensed health care givers with the authority to prescribe are needed in other states that may not necessarily be in their jurisdiction. Various legal provisions ensure that health care givers are deployed in the affected state and they are given temporal practice permits as well as all the equipment and help they need for a conducive work environment. As soon as a state governor declares an emergency, reciprocity laws are activated and certain licensure laws are waivered.

The EMAC which stands for the Emergency Management Assistant Compact allows the licensed health care givers from one state to offer their health care services to the state that is faced with an emergency. The care givers have the authority to write prescriptions that are consistent with all terms of a health care giver licensure. EMAC only works in local government and state agents so it is possible for a nurse working in a local health facility to be covered under EMAC while a physician from a private hospital is not.

Many states are increasingly enacting laws that allow them to provide health care services outside their state of jurisdiction during an emergency. So far, over 14 states have adopted a part of the Model State Emergency Health Powers Act that waivers all licensure requirements during a declared emergency for care givers who are serving in that affected state if they are licensed back in their states. On top of that, UEVHPA allows volunteer health providers who are registered to provide their services through local host institutions during an emergency.

Both UEVHPA and MSEHPA provide all that is needed for the health care givers during and after the emergency. Mental health care givers who have the authority to prescribe medication are allowed to fully practice in the affected state. Federal health workers who are licensed in their states are allowed to work in any of the federal facilities like a VA hospital before and after an emergency which makes it easier for them to reach the affected populations.

Provisions, emergency laws and compacts such as MSEHPA, UEVHPA and EMAC have civil liability protection laws for the health care givers who go to serve in another state during an emergency. These protections deal even with prescribing authority. If you are a physician who has prescription authority back at home, then you are protected by the liability protection when you prescribe medication in the host state. However some reciprocity provisions demand that visiting nurses should practice in accordance to the host state's law. If you have prescribing authority in your home state but a host state bares physicians from prescribing, then the liability protection law cannot cover you.

Mental healthcare givers are required to always follow the state and federal laws that govern the prescribing of drugs even during emergencies whether the care givers are providing services in their states or host states. The state and federal laws contain very few emergency provisions that enable dispensing and prescribing of drugs such as psychotropic drugs to patients who depend on the drugs to manage chronic mental illness. A good example is the federal law that states that under normal circumstances drugs under schedule 2 should only be given through an authorized written prescription.

In the event that there is an emergency and a patient is required to take a certain dosage of a controlled substance under schedule 2 and no other alternative medication is available, then the prescriber can verify without doubt that the only solution is to provide the medication, then give that particular medication but only the required dosage and not more.

# Chapter 7: How to Interpret Medical Orders

It is important for nurses, technicians and any other medical personnel to understand how to interpret medical orders provided a physician, because it is the only way to ascertain the patient receives the treatment found to be fitting. Such proficiency also ensures no medical errors are caused in the course of providing treatment for the patient.

A lot of important medical information is given in very short form, and everyone involved in treating a patient needs to understand the language involved. Part of the language is in form of abbreviations, and so this part of the book will deal with medical abbreviations commonly used in the medical field.

### *Medical Abbreviations Commonly Used*

Many medical abbreviations are found in matters of pertaining to dosage and administration of drugs, a good number appearing in prescriptions as well as clients' charts. Some of the abbreviations are actually in Latin, but the important thing is to know what each term or short form represents as far as matters of medication are concerned, and to be prepared to use that correct meaning consistently.

In this chapter, you will see some abbreviations commonly used in the administration of medication and others used to indicate the various routes by which medication is administered. Still others are indication of the form of dosage. You will particularly learn about various symbols commonly used as well as abbreviations commonly used to indicate varying measurement units.

### *Medication Related Abbreviations*

1. a.c. in the field of medicine denotes before food.

2. a.m.

3. a.m. denotes before noon.

4. aa. denotes of each

5.

6. Ad

Ad is written in prescriptions as it is, and it essentially means up to. It is used to basically denote a limit.

7. Ad libitum

Ad libitum is abbreviated as 'ad lib', and it means freely or at the person's pleasure. It means no limit has been given for the particular product and so the person can consume as much as they desire.

8. alt.

alt. represents alternate

9. alt. die

alt. die stands for alternate days.

10. amp

amp denotes ampoule, which is a glass capsule that holds an amount of liquid meant for an injection.

11. Ana

Ana, a term abbreviated as ăă, means of each.

12. Ante

Ante is another medical term used often in medical dosing, and it is abbreviated as 'a', and its actual meaning is before.

13. Ante cibum

Ante cibum is abbreviated in medicine as a.c. and its meaning is before meals. This means any medication dose accompanied by this abbreviation portrays the importance of the patient taking the medication before feeding.

14. applic.

applic. stands for apply

15. aq. / aqua

aq. or even aqua denotes water

16. aur.

   aur denotes ear

17. aurist

   aurist simply means eardrops

18. Bene

   Bene is abbreviated as 'ben', and its meaning is well or good.

19. b.

   b. in the medical field is an abbreviation for twice.

20. b.d.

   b.d. is also used to mean two times on a daily basis.

21. b.i.d.

   b.i.d. is also used to denote two times in a day every day.

22. Bis

   Bis is written as it is and it means twice.

23. Bis in die

   'Bis in die' as a medical term is abbreviated as b.i.d. The meaning of this term is two times a day.

24. c.

   c. in the medical field is an abbreviation meaning 'with'.

25. calid.

   'calid' used in the medical field acts as an abbreviation for 'warm'.

26. cap.

   cap. is an abbreviation for capsule

27. cib.

cib. is an abbreviation for food.

28. co.

co. in the medical field denotes 'compound'.

29. collut.

In the medical field, 'collut.' is used to denote 'mouthwash'.

30. collyr.

collyr. in the medical field represents eye lotion.

31. conc.

conc. is simply an abbreviation for 'concentrated'.

32. crem.

crem. is used as an abbreviation for cream.

33. Capiat

Capiat, when used as a medical term is abbreviated as 'Cap, and it means *'let the client take'*.

34. Capsula

Capsula, when used as a medical term, is abbreviated as 'caps', and its meaning is capsule.

35. d.

In the medical field 'd.' is an abbreviation for 'a day'.

36. Dentur

'Dentur tales doses' is a medical term abbreviated as D.T.D. or d.t.d., and it means *'give of such doses'*.

37. dest.

dest. is used in the medical field as abbreviation for 'distilled'.

38. dil.

dil. is used in the medical field as abbreviation for 'diluted'.

39. Dispensa

   Dispensa is abbreviated as 'Disp', and its meaning is simply 'dispense'.

40. div.

   div. is used in the medical field as abbreviation for 'divide'.

41. dol.urg.

   dol.urg is an abbreviation used to denote 'the time when pain is severe'.

42. dolent.part

   dolent.part is an abbreviation used in the medical field to denote 'to the part that is afflicted'.

43. dos.

   In the medical field 'dos.' is used as abbreviation for dose.

44. et

   et is used in the medical field as it is and its meaning is simply 'and'.

45. ex modo praescripto

   'ex modo praescripto' is abbreviated as e.m.p., and its meaning is after the manner prescribed or directed.

46. ex aq.

   ex aq. is used as abbreviation for 'in water'.

47. ext.

   ext. in the medical field is abbreviation for 'extract'.

48. extemp.

   'extemp.' in the medical field is an abbreviation for 'extemporaneously dispensed'.

49. Fac/fiat/fiant

fac/fiat/fiant have their abbreviations in the medical language as 'ft'.

The meaning they represent is either 'make' or 'let it be made'.

50. fort.

'fort.' is used in the medical field as abbreviation for 'strong'.

51. garg.

'garg.' is used as abbreviation for 'gargle'.

52. gtt./guttae

'gtt.' or 'guttae' is an abbreviation used in the medical field to denote 'drops'.

53. Granum

Granum, used in the medical field, is abbreviated as 'gr.', and it simply means grain.

54. Gutta/Guttae

Gutta/Guttae is abbreviated as either 'gt' or 'gtt', and the meaning is either drop or drops.

55. h.

h. is an abbreviation for 'at the hour of'.

56. h.s.

h.s. is used as abbreviation for at the time of going to bed/bedtime.

57. Hora

Hora is abbreviated as 'hor' or simply 'h', and in the medical language it means 'hour'.

58. Hora somni

Hora somni is abbreviated as 'hor som' or 'h.s.', and it means 'at the hour of sleep'.

59. i.c.

i.c. is an abbreviation used in the medical field to denote 'between meals'.

60. IM

IM is an abbreviation used in the medical field to denote 'intramuscular'.

61. inf

'inf' is an abbreviation used in the medical field to denote 'infusion'.

62. inj

'inj' is an abbreviation used in the medical field to denote 'injection'.

63. IV

IV in the medical field is an abbreviation used to denote 'intravenous'.

64. Injectio

Injectio is abbreviated as 'inj' and it simply means injection.

65. Inter

Inter is used as it is, and its meaning is simply 'between'.

66. Lotio

Lotio is abbreviated as 'lot', and it simply means lotion.

67. m./mane

m. or mane, used in the medical field, is an abbreviation for 'morning time'.

68. m.d.

m.d. is an abbreviation used in the medical field to denote 'as directed'.

69. m.d.u.

m.d.u. is an abbreviation for 'to be used as directed'.

70. MDI

MDI is used as abbreviation for 'metered dose inhaler'.

71. mist.

mist. as used in the medical field denotes 'mixture'.

72. mitt./mitte

mitt. or mitte is used as an abbreviation in the medical field denoting 'send'.

73. n./nocte

n. or nocte, when used in the medical field, is an abbreviation for 'during the night'.

74. n.et m.

n.et m. is used in the medical field as abbreviation for 'both night and morning'.

75. narist.

narist. simply means 'nasal drops' in the medical field.

76. NP/n.p.

Either NP or n.p. in the medical language is an abbreviation denoting 'proper name'.

77. Non repetatur

Non repetatur is abbreviated as either 'non rep' or 'non repetat', and the meaning it bears is 'do not repeat'.

78. o.alt.hor

o.alt.hor. is an abbreviation used in the medical field to denote 'every other hour'.

79. o.d.

In the medical field, o.d. is an abbreviation for 'everyday'.

80. o.m.

o.m. is an abbreviation that denotes 'every morning' in the medical field.

81. o.n.

o.n. in the medical field is an abbreviation for 'every night'.

82. oculent.

oculent. in the medical field denotes 'eye ointment'.

83. Octarius

Octarius is abbreviated as 'O.' and its meaning is pint.

84. Oculus dexter

Oculus dexter is abbreviated as 'O.D.', and its meaning in the medical language is 'right eye'.

85. Oculus sinister

Oculus sinister is abbreviated as either 'o.s' or 'O.S.', and its meaning in the medical language is 'left eye'.

86. Oculi unitas

Oculi unitas is abbreviated as 'O.U.', and its meaning is 'both eyes'.

87. Omni hora

Omni hora is abbreviated as 'Omni.hor.', and its meaning is 'every hour'.

88. p.a.

p.a. is used in the medical field as abbreviation for 'to the affected part'.

89. p.aeq.

p.aeq. is used in the medical field as abbreviation denoting 'equal parts'.

90. p.c.

p.c. is used in the medical field as abbreviation for 'after food.

91. p.m.

p.m. is used as abbreviation for afternoon

92. p.r.n.

p.r.n. is used to denote 'when needed'.

93. part. dolent.

part. dolent. in the medical field stands for 'to the painful part'.

94. past.

past. in the medical field is used to denote 'paste'.

95. PR

PR is an abbreviation used in the medical field to represent 'per rectum'.

96. pulv.

pulv. used in the medical field is abbreviation for powder.

97. PV

PV is used as abbreviation in the medical field to denote 'per vagina'.

98. Per

Per is used as it is to mean either through or by means of.

99. Per os/P.O.

'Per os' or P.O. means 'by mouth'

100.    Placebo

Placebo is used as it is and its meaning is 'I will satisfy'.

101.    Post cibum

Post cibum is abbreviated as 'post cib' or 'p.c.', and its meaning is after meals or as needed, or even as circumstances require.

102.    Pulvis

Pulvis is abbreviated as 'pulv' and its meaning is powder.

103.    q.d.

q.d. in the medical field represents 'four times on a daily basis'.

104.    q.d.s.

q.d.s. in medical terms is an abbreviation for 'to be taken four times every day'.

105.    q.q.h.

q.q.h. means 'every 4$^{th}$ hour'.

106.   q.s.

q.s. is an abbreviation for 'sufficient'.

107.   q12h

q12h is an abbreviation denoting 'every twelve hours'.

108.   q4h

q4h is an abbreviation denoting 'every four hours'.

109.   q6h

q6h is an abbreviation denoting 'every six hours'.

110.   qq.

qq. in medical terms is an abbreviation denoting 'every'.

111.   Quantum salts

'Quantum salts' is abbreviated as 'q.s.' and its meaning is 'a sufficient quantity'.

112.   Quantum salts ad

'Quantum salts ad' is abbreviated as 'q.s ad' and its meaning is 'a sufficient quantity to make'.

113.   Quaque

Quaque is abbreviated as 'q.' and it means every.

114.   Quaque die

'Quaque die' is abbreviated as 'q.d.' and its meaning is every day.

115.   Quaque hora

'Quaque hora' is abbreviated as 'q.h.' and its meaning is every hour.

116.   Quarter in die

'Quarter in die' is abbreviated as 'q.i.d.' and its meaning is 'four times a day'.

Recipe as a medical term is abbreviated as 'Rx', and means 'take thou'.

117. Rx

Rx as an abbreviation is the medical field means 'take'.

118. Semi, semis

'Semi, semis' when used as a medical term, is abbreviated as 'ss' and it means a half.

119. signa

'signa' is abbreviated as 'sig' and its meaning is either write or label.

120. Sine

'Sine' in the medical field is abbreviated simply as 's' and it means without.

121. s.o.s.

In medical terms, the abbreviation, s.o.s. means 'if necessary'.

122. SC

SC is used as an abbreviation in the medical field to denote 'subcutaneous'.

123. SL

SL is used as an abbreviation in the medical field to denote 'sublingual'.

124. Solve/Solvere/Solutus

Solve/Solvere/Solutus are word choices used in the medical field and abbreviated as 'solv', and they bear the meaning of 'dissolve'.

125. Statim

'Statim' is abbreviated as 'stat', and in the medical field it means immediately.

126. Tabella

'Tabella' is another term used in the medical field and abbreviated as 'tab', and it simply means tablet.

127. Ter

'Ter' has its abbreviation as 't.', and its meaning is three.

128. Ter in die

'Ter in die' is abbreviated as 't.i.d.' or 'tid', and it means three times a day.

129. t.d.d.

t.d.d. is another abbreviation used to denote 'three times every day'.

130. t.d.s.

t.d.s. is used as an abbreviation in the medical field to denote 'to be taken three times every day'.

131. tinct.

tinct. is used to mean 'tincture'.

132. trit./triturate

'trit.' or 'triturate' is used in the medical field to stand for 'serial dilution or mixing of ingredients'.

133. u.a.

In medical terms, 'u.a.' is used to denote 'as before'.

134. Unguentum

'Unguentum' is abbreviated as 'ung' and its meaning is 'an ointment'.

135. Ut dictum

'Ut dictum' is abbreviated as 'Ut dict.' and its meaning is 'as directed'.

136. WSP

WSP is used as an abbreviation to denote 'white soft paraffin'.

137. YSP

YSP is used as an abbreviation in the medical field to denote 'yellow soft paraffin'.

### The Apothecary Abbreviation System

The abbreviations in the apothecary abbreviation system pertain to weight and volume, and despite this system having come into use centuries ago, it is still in common use. Within this apothecary system, the smallest unit in weight is the grain and the smallest in volume is referred to as minim. When grain is written in short form, its abbreviation is never written in capital letters – it is always written as 'gr'.

The term, apothecary' was assimilated into the English language during the 14<sup>th</sup> century, having been derived from the Latin word, *apothēca,* which means a storehouse. In its early use, the term was used in reference to a person skilled in preparation of medicines, whom in modern day is the pharmacist.

### Weight & Volume Abbreviations

(1) Milligram is abbreviated as 'mg'

(2) Gram is abbreviated as 'gr' or simply 'g'.

(3) Kilogram is abbreviated as either 'kg' or 'Kg'

(4) Grain is abbreviated as 'gr'

(5) Dram is abbreviated as '3'

(6) Ounce is abbreviated as 'oz'

(7) Milliliter is abbreviated as 'ml'

(8) Cubic centimeters is abbreviated as 'cc'

(9) Liter is abbreviated as either 'l' or 'L'.

(10)    fluid dram is abbreviated as f3

(11)    fluid ounce is abbreviated as fl.oz  or f3

(12)    pint is abbreviated as pt.

(13)    Quart is abbreviated as qt

(14)    gallon is abbreviated as gal.

When it comes to the fluid dram and the fluid ounce, often their abbreviations are without the 'f'. This is because there is an assumption that the symbol of dram used in cases of a liquid bears the intended use of 'fluid dram'.

## Abbreviations Relating to Administration of Medication

(1) P.O. is used to denote 'by mouth'.

(2) I.D. is used to denote 'intradermal'.

(3) I.M. is used to denote 'intramuscular'.

(4) I.V. is used to denote 'intravenous'

(5) S.C. is used to denote 'subcutaneous'.

(6) T.D. is used to denote 'transdermal'.

## Abbreviations Discouraged in the Medical Field

(1) 'u' should not be used to denote 'unit' to avoid the risk of it being read as a zero.

(2) 'IV' should not be used to denote 'International Units' lest it be confused for 10.

(3) Q.D. or QD, or even q.d. or qd should not be used to denote 'daily' as it is sometimes causes confusion when being read.

(4) Q.O.D. or QOD, or even q.o.d. or qod should not be used to stand for 'every other day' for the same reason of causing confusion when being read.

(5) .x mg is discouraged from use as an abbreviation for O.X. mg, because sometimes medical staff members overlook the decimal point.

(6) MS, an abbreviation that stands for Morphine sulfate, is discouraged for fear it might be confused for magnesium sulfate.

(7) $MSO_4$, which is used as abbreviation for Morphine sulfate, is discouraged for use because it can be easily confused for magnesium sulfate that is rightly abbreviated as $MgSO_4$.

(8) $MgSO_4$ is also discouraged for use to avoid confusion with morphine sulfate ($MSO_4$).

It has also been noted that decimals can cause confusion when information is being transferred from the medication record, and so their use is discouraged. For example, if a doctor means to write point three milligrams and so writes .3mg, a nurse may miss out the decimal and end up confusing that measure of dose to be 3mg. Obviously, this would result in a big discrepancy in the dosage and may cause medical problems for the patient. To avoid such confusion, medical practitioners are encouraged to begin measures of small doses with a zero, what is usually described as a leading zero. So, in case of point three milligrams the doctor would write it as 0.3mg. Such a measure shows at a glance that it is below a whole unit; the measure is outright in decimals.

It has also been noted that decimals can also cause confusion when used with whole numbers, so whenever they can be left out without making a difference in the measure of dosage they are best left out. A good example is when a doctor wants to write two milligrams and so writes in the medication record, 2.0mg. It is easy for the nurse or other medical staff to confuse that measure for 20mg, which would lead to overdosing a patient. For that reason, whenever the measure is a whole number, it is best left as it is without a decimal point. In our example here, instead of writing 2.0mg the doctor is advised to write simply 2mg.

Of course if there is a decimal above a whole number that would be different and using a decimal in such cases causes no confusion whatsoever. For instance, two point five milligrams can be written as 2.5mg without causing any confusion. In any case, the decimal of a measure has to be represented in the measure.

Good news is that many health institutions in present day have established CPOE systems, and so there is rarely need for the nurse to transfer information manually. This means chances of the doctor's instructions in the medical record being misinterpreted due to the writing are minimal.

### *Roman Numerals in Medicine*

Roman numerals happen to be in common use when it comes to writing of prescriptions. Their use is often indication of the precise amount of medicinal ingredients contained in the product, if the system being used is the one referred to as apothecary system. You will also see the Roman numerals used in specifying the medicinal units that require dispensing, for example, the number of capsules or tablets, or even units of powders or suppositories and so on.

By the end of this chapter, you will be able to tell what it means when the doctor writes in Roman numerals, for example, 'Dispxv'. These numerals are also used in the signa, where a signature is put just before making out the prescription, and the nurse or any other medical personnel using the prescription should be in a position to understand how the Roman numerals system works within the field of pharmacy.

### Basic Roman Symbols

I, which in its origin means 'unus', stands for one or 1

V, which in its origin means 'quinque', stands for five or 5

X, which in its origin means 'decem,' stands for ten or 10

L, which in its origin means 'quiquaginta', stands for fifty or 50

C, which in its origin means 'centum', stands for a hundred or 100

D, which in its origin means 'quingenti', stands for five hundred or 500

M, which in its origin means 'mille', stands for a thousand or 1000

It is correct to state that the entire system of Roman numerals comprises just seven letters, and all other quantities are formed from combinations of letters chosen from these basic seven. These letters are in Latin.

Once you are conversant with these basic symbols, you can form wide ranging combinations, all representing different measures. In short, the numbers not represented in the above list are numerous and you need them in prescriptions, but you can create them using these few basic symbols provided. However, to be proficient in writing or understanding Roman numbers, you need to understand the rules guiding their formation.

There are times, and more so when writing medical prescriptions, when the end of a Roman number is marked by a 'j' as in 'iij'. In such an instance, the 'j' will be holding the position of an 'i', since the number intended is 'iii' or simply 'three'. Another good example is number 7 written in Roman, which ordinarily is 'vii', but this time the last 'i' is substituted with a 'j'. Number 7 in Roman hence becomes 'vij'. The origin of this use of 'j' was an effort to deter forgery. Once a number had a 'j' at the end, there was no way of adding another numeral as putting a 'j' in that position marked the end of the number as intended and written by the original writer.

### Repetition in Writing Roman Numerals

Sometimes certain numerals are repeated in writings within the medical field, and in such instances, it means the value represented by those numerals is also repeated. This is particularly so when Roman numerals are in use. So, considering that X represents 10,

X repeated as in XXX means the number represents 10+10+10, which totals 30. As for C, having a repeating C as in CC simply means the value of C counted twice. C in Roman numerals stands for a hundred, and so CC means 100+100 and that totals 200.

In fact repetition is a tool used to create Roman numbers not represented by the seven major ones already introduced, and when it is not a matter of repetition then it is a matter of combining one or more of the original seven Roman numerals.

Number 2 is hence represented by a repeated 'i' to become 'ii' while 3 is represented by 'i' repeated three times to become 'iii'. As for number 4, it is a combination of 'i' and 'v', where as earlier explained the value of 'i' is subtracted from the value of 'v' to produce the value, 4. So, four is written as 'iv'; six as 'vi'; seven as 'vii'; eight as 'viii'; and nine as 'ix'.

When it comes to number eleven, 'i' is added to 'x' to produce 'xi'. You just need to think in terms of the value ten added the value of one. When using addition, the numeral with the smaller value is put on the right side of the one with a bigger value. Along this same line of thinking, you have number twenty-two being written as the numerals comprising 20 added the numerals representing 2. The end result is xxii.

As for combinations involving both additions and subtractions, a good example is 41, where it is best to think in terms of the numerals for 40 added the numeral for 1. In this case there will be 'xl', as 10 is subtracted from 50, and then 'i' will be added. In short, forty-one as a Roman number is either XLI or xli.

### *How to Write Massive Numbers as Roman Numerals*

When it comes to numbers that are as massive as 4,000 and even more, the tendency is to add a bar above a given base numeral, and positioning of such a bar denotes the need to multiply that numeral by 1,000.

As such,

$\overline{V}$ represents 5,000, which comes from 5 x 1,000.

$\overline{X}$ represents 10,000, which comes from 10 x 1,000.

$\overline{L}$ represents 50,000, which comes from 50 x 1,000.

$\overline{C}$ represents 100,000, which comes from 100 x 1,000.

$\overline{D}$ represents 500,000, which comes from 500 x 1,000.

$\overline{M}$ represents 1,000,000, which comes from 1,000 x 1,000.

### How to Write Very Big Numbers as Roman Numerals

When the number you want to write is massively huge, such as in millions, there is a way of writing them in Roman and keeping the numeral short and uncomplicated. The tendency is to underline the base numeral or to put some double bar below the numeral. Following this guide, it is easy to see that five million/5,000,000 can be written as an underlined V to become V̲, or as a V with a double bar at the bottom to become V̲.

If it is a case of 20,000,000, obviously, the base numeral will be taken to be 20, which in Roman is XX, and then that base numeral is either underlined or given a double bar at the bottom to become either XX̲ or XX̲.

### Rules Guiding Calculations Involving Roman Numerals

Rule No. 1 is that any time there is a letter, or even more than one letter, following a letter with greater value, the value of that last letter ought to be added to the bigger value.

For example, if you have C followed by X and then followed by I, meaning you have CXI, it is clear that I follows a letter with greater value that itself, X, while that X also follows a letter that beats it in value, C. The value represented by the Roman number, CXI, can be viewed as 100 + 10 + 1, as C means 100, X means 10 and I means 1.

100 + 10 + 1 = 111, and so the value of CXI is simply 111

Rule No. 2 is that if you have a letter placed to the left of a letter that is of greater value than itself, then the value of the number on the left side is subtracted from the greater value.

A good example is if you have X placed to the left of C. Since the value of X is 10 and that of C is a hundred, XC means the value of X subtracted from the value of C; and the result constitutes the value of XC.

XC = 100 − 10

XC = 90

Rule No. 3 takes into account that when using Roman numerals you can have a number made up of several letters; three, four, five, or even more letters. The easiest way to figure out the value represented by the entire range of Roman numerals is to first of all subtract the values that need to be subtracted, as explained in Rule No. 2, and then to deal with the addition as explained in Rule No. 1.

For example, if you have CCXIX, you will notice that the letters in CCX all have their values in descending order, which means none of the Roman numerals has a smaller value to its left. So that bit of the number is supposed to be left as it is first. However, the last part of the number needs subtraction, because the value of X is greater than the value of I that is to the left.

In short, when you see CCXIX, the first step should be to split the cluster that does not require subtraction and the one that requires subtraction. You will, therefore, have:

CCX + (IX)

After working on IX, which is 10 − 1, you will be left with CCX + (9)

You can now add the value of the letters, CCX, and then proceed to add 9.

CCX + 9 = 100 + 100 + 10 + 9 = 219

So, by doing the subtraction first and then doing the addition, it has been established that CCXIX = 219.

Rule No. 4 states that although it is fine to have a letter used in Roman calculations repeated within a given Roman number, such repetition should not exceed three times. Consider this: When writing 8 as a Roman number, the letter I is repeated three times after the letter V. In short, number 8 is written as VIII. One might expect number 9 to be written as number 8 but have I added to it so that you have VIIII, but this is against the convention of Roman numerals. For that reason, number 9 is written as (10 − 1), which is IX.

Another good example is CCC, the number that is actually 300. If you want to write 400, it is not allowed that you add another C to make a fourth. Instead, you move ahead and get the number representing 500 and then you subtract 100. That is the reason 400 is written in Roman as CD. D represents 500 and when you subtract 100 you get 400.

Rule number 5 is about exceptions to the rules already listed, and it involves the letters, V and L as well as D. For starters you never subtract these to create a new Roman number as in the two examples just shown. Also, these three Roman numerals do not get repeated. This means you cannot write VVV and call that 15 or write LL and call that 100. Even DD will not suffice for the value, one thousand.

When you want to write 15 you just write X that represents 10 and then add the V whose value is 5. In short number 15 is written in Roman as XV. For a hundred, as has already been noted, C is the letter to use. When you want to write 1,000, you have M to use.

### The Upper and Lower Case

In the system of Roman numbers, it is matters if the letter is in the upper or lower case. Many physicians, when making out their prescriptions, have a preference for the uppercase, but when it comes to writing 'I' as a small letter, they simply put a dot above it. Here below are the major rules that ought to be followed when writing medical prescriptions using Roman numerals.

### About Fractions

Whenever a measure is given in a medical prescription, Arabic numerals are used. Arabic numerals are those numbers represented by 0, 1, 2 all the way to 9. The only exception to this rule is when the measure is in reference to a half, which one might anticipate the use of 1/2, but which in the field of medicine is represented by 'ss'. Sometimes the 'ss' comes with a bar so that it appears as '–ss'. Otherwise all other fractions in medical prescriptions are in Arabic numerals. For example, a quarter would be written as 1/4, a third as 1/3 and so on.

# Chapter 8: How to Interpret Drug Orders

Doctors writing prescriptions ordinarily make use of the abbreviations already explained in the book, and more to be explained as you proceed, and so the people meant to use those prescriptions need to have the knowledge about such abbreviations. They especially need to be equipped with the skills to do the necessary calculations so that the prescription is executed as stipulated, and the patients benefit from the medical drugs as anticipated.

In short, the nurse charged with giving the doses written in the prescription needs to be in a position to read the doctor's orders as written; meaning with total accuracy. It is also important to know the measure equivalents, so that if the doctor writes the medication order in units different from those on the pharmacy drugs the nurse and any other concerned medical personnel can know how to calculate the correct dose to administer to the patient.

### *A Table Useful in Dosage Conversions*

ImL or milliliter = 1 cc or 1 cubic centimeter

1tsp or teaspoon = 5mL or milliliters

1,000mL or milliliters = 1L or liter

1tbsp or tablespoon =3tsp or teaspoons

1mg or milligram = 1,000mcg or micrograms

1oz or ounce = 2tbsp or tablespoon

1kg or kilogram = 1,000g or grams

1oz or ounce = 30mL or milliliters

1g or gram = 1,000mg or milligrams

1kg or kilogram = 2.2lb or pounds

1tbsp or tablespoon = 15mL or milliliters

### Abbreviated Doctor's Orders Exemplified

(a) The doctor has written: Tab iii stat, then tab ii bid

The correct interpretation of this order is: Three tablets once, then two tablets two times a day.

(b) The doctor has written: Tsp i pc & hs

The correct interpretation of this order is: One teaspoonful after meals and also at bedtime.

(c) The doctor has written: 3 ml IM stat & q24h

The correct interpretation for this order is: Three milliliters intramuscularly at once and thereafter every 24 hours.

(d) The doctor has written: Tab iii stat, then tab i q4h

The correct interpretation for the doctor's order is: Three tablets at once and then one tablet after every four hours.

In fact, among the abbreviations nurses and other medical staff should master are those associated with the frequency of medication administration. If the medication record shows medication should be administered after every hour, administering the medication after ten hours would render the doctor's prescription useless. On the other hand, if the medication record indicates the medication should be administered after ten hours, administering the medication after one hour would be a big risk and might jeopardize the health of the patient.

Among the factors doctors consider in prescribing certain times as well as frequency for administration of medication, are the rate at which the particular medication is absorbed into the body, possible medication side effects, possibility of the medication interacting with some other prescribed medication, and the results the doctor anticipates after the patient has had the medication.

Normally, times of administering medication to in-patients is fixed, with there being a hospital policy guiding the particular hours for giving medication to patients. For example, in some hospitals it is well known that at 6pm nurses are expected to be going round giving medications. Another round may come at midnight. Ordinarily medical practitioners prescribing medication just indicate the frequency by which the patient should take particular medication, and it is up to the hospital to fix the exact hours to deliver the medication. For the institutions using the eMAR system, the practitioner could do prescription using CPOE and the regularity is organized by the computerized system.

### *Abbreviations Specific to Medication Administration Frequency*

'a' is used to denote 'before'.

'a.c.' is used to denote 'before meals'.

'b.i.d.'/bid is used to represent 'two times a day'.

'b.i.w.' stands for 'two times in a week'.

'h'/'hr' is short for 'hour'.

'h.s.' is abbreviation for 'hour of sleep' or 'bedtime'

'min' stands for 'minute'.

'noc'/'noct' stands for 'during the night'.

'o.n.' is an abbreviation for 'every night'.

'p' stands for 'after'.

'p.c.' is abbreviation for 'after meals'.

'q' stands for 'each' or 'every'.

'q.a.m.' stands for 'every morning'.

'q.h.' / 'qh' stands for 'every hour'.

'qXh' is abbreviation for 'every X hours, with 'X' standing for any given number of hours'

'q.h.s.'/ 'qhs' represents 'every night at bedtime'.

'stat'/ 'STAT' means 'immediately' / 'at once'

't.i.d.' / 'tid' stands for '3 times in a day'.

't.i.w.' stands for '3 times in a week'.

PRN represents 'as needed'.

### Understanding the PRN

It is important to remember that prescriptions are given within some context and corresponding dosage calculations then follow, and such context is the reason some additional information is provided in this book, over and beyond math. It is in this light that nurses and other medical personnel involved in medication administration need to understand what a PRN is and its significance in the entire process of patient care.

A PRN can be described as that order that the doctor issues to instruct the nurse concerned to give the patient medication as per the patient's need, a need that the prescribing doctor will have established before defining the criteria to be followed in administering the medication.

As for the criteria the doctor follows, these are essentially parameters comprising the patient's ranges of pain, blood pressure or even temperature. As already mentioned, the medication order must be complete by the time it gets to the nurse for use.

### How to Tackle Dosage Problems

In order to tackle a problem of dosage properly, there are some steps you need to follow, and the first one is defining the actual problem that needs resolving. For example, is the problem about finding out the amount of medication the patient requires given the amount of medication in a single tablet? Such kinds of problems require calculating mass for mass, and there are some illustrations to follow in this chapter.

Other problems that you need to be able to calculate involve mass for liquid or even liquid for liquid. For example, given the amount of medication in a certain amount of liquid how much of the liquid should you give the patient? Examples will soon follow.

Other problems require that you be able to calculate the amount of IV to give a patient given the concentration of medication in a given volume. Other times it is the rate the nurse and other medical staff are required to calculate when provided with the amount of liquid the patient needs and the time it should take to administer it.

Other times you would need to calculate the dosage you need to administer to the patient given the dosage that corresponds to a certain body weight. Such problems are usually common when the patient is a child.

### How to Convert Dosing Units involving Mass

When you are required to convert micrograms to milligrams; milligrams to grams; grams to kilograms; which in abbreviations is mcg to mg; mg to g; and g to kg; all you need to do is divide the units you have by 1,000.

When you want to do the reverse, which is converting kilograms to grams; grams to milligrams; or even milligrams to micrograms; you just need to multiply the units you have by 1,000.

### Illustration: Conversion of Micrograms to Milligrams

Convert 7,000 mcg to mg

All you need to do is divide the value you have in mcg by 1,000 in order to find the value in mg. In this case, calculate 7,000mcg ÷ 1,000 and you will get 7mg.

In cases where you are required to convert mass from the imperial units of measure to the metric units of measure, such as pounds to kilograms, whose abbreviation is lb to kg, you need to divide the units you have by 2.2.

When the converse is required of you, meaning you need to convert units of mass given in metric terms to imperial units of measure, such as kilograms to lbs, you need to multiply the units you have by 2.2.

### Illustration: Conversion of Pounds to Kilograms

Convert 55lb to kg.

All you need to do is take the value you have in pounds and divide it by 2.2 in order to find out what the value will be in kilograms. In this case, calculate 55lb ÷ 2.2 and the answer will be 25kg.

### How to Convert Dosing Units involving Volume

When there is need to convert microliters to milliliters; milliliters to litres; and from liters to kiloliters; which in abbreviations is mcL to mL; mL to L; and L to kL; you need to divide by 1,000. If the conversion is in the reverse, meaning you want to convert kiloliters to liters; liters to milliliters; and from milliliters to microliters; you just need to multiply the figure you have by 1,000.

### Illustration: Conversion of Liters to Microliters

Convert 0.005 L to mcL.

What you need to do convert the value you have in liters to the value in microLiters is to first multiply what you have by 1,000 in order to find the value in milliliters, and then convert the milliliters into microLiters by multiplying that value by 1,000. In this case, calculate 0.005L x 1,000 and you will get 5mL.

Then calculate 5mL x 1,000 and you will get 5,000mcL.

### How to Convert Dosing Units involving Time

When you need to convert minutes to hours

In converting values in minutes to values in hours, you need to divide what you have by 60, and when you want to convert a value in hours into a value in minutes you simply multiply what you have by 60.

Illustration: Conversion of Hours to Minutes

Convert 6hr to min.

To find out the number of minutes in 6 hours, meaning to convert the 6 hours you have into minutes, calculate 6hr x 60 and you will get 360min.

### How to Convert Dosing Units Involving Mass

In case all you have been given is some mass, how to do you convert that mass into tablets in order to give to the patient?

The method to follow is taking the mass given in the medication order and to divide it by the mass that makes up one tablet according to the packaging. What you get as your answer constitutes the number of tablets you need to give the patient. The formula is given as:

Mass in the Order / Mass Available= Number of tablets to be given

### Illustration: Calculation of Tablets when Mass Ordered differs from Available

The medication, Metoprolol, which is the drug contained in brands like Lopressor, has been ordered, and the medication order reads 25mg PO. The medication supplied to the hospital is in 50mg tablets. How do you find out the number of tablets of the mass you have to give to the patient?

The way to find out the number of tablets of 50mg to give the patient in order to adhere to the medication order is to take the mass ordered and to divide it by the mass available. The result you get constitutes the number of tablets you need to give the patient. The easiest way to do this calculation is:

25mg/50mg= ½ tablet

### *Illustration on Calculation on No. of Tablets to Dispense*

Suppose the doctor orders the patient to be given 40mg of Potassium Chloride, such as the drug contained in the brand, K-Dur, and the hospital has tablets in 10mg. How many of such 10mg tablets would the nurse need to give the patient?

The formula here remains the same, meaning what is ordered divided by what is available.

Mass in the Order / Mass Available = Number of tablets to be given

In this case, the calculation necessary would be:

40mg/10mg, and since 40 divided by 10 is 4 and the mg units would cancel out completely, the answer of 4 would represent 4 tablets; what the nurse should give the patient.

### *How to Convert Dosing Units involving Mass vs Liquid*

In case you are provided with the amount of mass in a given amount of liquid, and you need to give the patient the right amount of liquid, how do you go about finding out the amount of liquid to give?

What you do is take the amount issued in the medication order and divide the figure by the amount available, and then you multiply the result you get with the Volume of what you have.

Amount Ordered / Amount Available x Volume Per What is Available

If this sounds a little complex, you will find it easier when you see the illustration in real figures.

## Illustration: Calculation of Drug Proportion to Administer from Available

The doctor orders Phenytoin drug as contained in the brand, Dilantin, and the dose is 0.1g PO, with instructions to administer the drug via nasogastric tube. In the hospital, this drug is available as 30mg per 5mL. What amount of the drug available would the nurse be required to administer to the patient? The formula to follow is shown here below.

Amount of drug ordered / Amount of drug available x Volume in the drug available

One important point to note is the need to divide like terms. In this case the doctor made the order in grams but the nurse has within the hospital is in milligrams. So you need to convert the grams ordered into milligrams.

Converting 0.1 grams to milligrams requires that you multiply 0.1g x 1,000, and the answer is 100mg. The calculation to establish the amount the patient ought to receive is:

100mg/30mg x 5mL

You can begin by canceling 5mL against 30mg, and when you do that using 5 as the common divisor, 5mL cancels out but leaves 1mL. 30mg divide by 5 produces 6mg. The units in mg accompanying the numerator and denominator also cancel out. At this juncture what you have is $\frac{100}{6}$ x 1mL.

Now multiply 100mg x 1mL and you will get 100mL, and once you put that over 6 you get the fraction, 100ml/6. The nurse will, therefore, need to administer to the patient 16.67 milliliters or 16.67mL of the available medication.

## Illustration to Calculate Medication Dose to Administer per IV Infusion

The doctor ordered the 40mg of the medication, Lasix, to be administered through IV. The drug the nurse has available is in 80m per one mL. How much of that available medication should the nurse draw up in readiness to administer? The formula to be used is the same one used in the previous illustration. It is:

Amount of drug ordered / Amount of drug available x Volume in the drug available

The calculation the nurse ought to do looks like this:

40mg/80mg x 1mL

The simplest start is to divide 40mg with 80mg, with their common divisor being 40mg. 40mg divided by 40mg has everything canceling out and the answer will be 1. In the meantime, dividing 80mg with 40mg has the units canceling out completely, and 80 divided by 40 produces 2. So the resultant fraction is:

½ x 1mL. In short, the nurse would need to administer to the patient half a milliliter of the available drug, which can be written as either ½ mL or 0.5mL.

When it comes to calculating medication dosage to be administered through IV, there are some basic ideas that need to be understood and adhered to. You need, for example, to understand the important terms used in relation to IV, and to be able to work with them as the doctor writing the medication record intended.

### *Crucial Terms & Abbreviations relating to IV Medication Administration*

1. 'gtts'

   'gtts' stands for drops

2. Drop factor

   The 'drop factor' is used in reference to the number of drops in a given mass of IV fluid. The drop factor, whose measurement is in gtts/mL, varies according to the type of tubing in use.

3. Flow Rate

   Flow rate is the measure used in reference to how the liquid is flowing through an IV. The measurement used for the flow rate is in gtts per minute (gtts/minute), or even in milliliters per hour (mL/hour). Ordinarily, the measure is given in gtts/minute when the IV is being regulated manually, whereas when it is being administered via some electronic regulator it is given in mL/hour.

4. D

   D, in relation to IV administration means Dextrose.

5. W

   In the administration of IV, W stands for water.

6. S stands for saline.

7. NS

   NS stands for normal saline, which is essentially 0.9%NaCl, where NaCl stands for Sodium Chloride.

8. RL/LR

The abbreviation, RL or even LR, when used in the context of administering IV, stands for 'Lactated Ringer's'.

<u>Illustration</u>

What does it mean when the doctor writes D5W?

D5W means you need to have 5% Dextrose in the water.

***Illustration to Decipher Doctor's Prescription***

What does it mean when the doctor writes D5 ¼ NS?

D5 ¼ NS means you need to have 5% Dextrose in 0.225% saline solution. Remember normal saline solution is 0.9% NaCl, and so if you divide 0.9 by 4 one quarter will be 0.225%.

***Determining Content in IV Fluids***

When a certain volume of IV fluid as well as dosage is put in form of percentage, how do you find out the mass of the given dosage? The formula is provided here below.

***How to Calculate Mass when provided with volume and dosage***

Concentration percentage /100 x Volume in mL = Amount of dosage in g

***Illustration to Calculate Dextrose Concentration in a Fluid***

Find out the dextrose amount within 1,000mL D5W.

Using the formula provided above, concentration percentage /100 x Volume in mL = Amount of dosage in g, it means:

5% / 100 x 1,000 mL = ? g

You can begin by canceling out the denominator, which is 100, where:

$100 \div 100 = 1$.

When you take the corresponding number as the 1,000mL across:

$1,000 \div 100 = 10$mL

So, at this point you have 5%/1 x 10 or 500/100 x 10

When next you solve 500/100 x 10, the first fraction can be simplified to 5/1, and so in whole what you have is 5/1 x 10.

5 x 10 = 50. Ignore the denominator, which is 1, as it makes no difference to the entire value. The answer is, therefore, 50g in every 1,000mL D5W.

Illustration

Find out the sodium chloride level within 2,000mL NS.

As you begin your calculation, it is important to remember that NS is consistently 0.9% NaCl.

So, using concentration percentage /100 x Volume in mL = Amount of dosage in g:

0.9%/100 x 2,000mL

If you cancel out the denominator, 100, and then divide the 2,000 by 100, you get 20. After this you will be looking at 0.9% of 20, which is essentially,( 0.9 x 100/100) x 20.

The result of that equation is 90/100x 20

 90/100x 20 = 1,800/100, which gives 18

In this illustration, 18g is the correct answer.

### *How to Calculate the Rate of IV Flow given Volume and Period*

When you have a set amount of liquid as well as a given time frame, what is the rate of IV flow in terms of mL/hr? The measurement used whenever the regulation of IV is done electronically using an infusion pump follows the formula here below.

volume in ml / time in hours. This is the formula that gives the IV rate of flow in mL/hr.

Illustration on Calculation of Flow Rate Given Volume & Time

If the instructions are that you infuse an amount of fluid, 250mL, over a period of 120 minutes using an infusion pump, you need to calculate the rate of flow as shown here below:

 volume in ml / time in hours, which in this case is 250ml/2hr

Notice you will have had to convert the minutes given into hours, and 120min converted to hours means 120÷60, which gives 2hrs.

250ml/2hr= 125ml/hr

### *Illustration: Calculation of Infusion Flow Rate Given Volume & Time*

The medication record had 1,000mL D5W IV ordered for infusion over a span of 10hrs, and the method of infusion was an infusion pump. As usual, the rate at which the medication should be infused should follow the formula:

Volume in ml / time in hours

In this case, the volume is 1,000mL and the period over which to do the infusion is 10hrs. The correct calculation is, therefore:

1,000ml /10hr, which gives 100mL/hr

### *Calculations Involving Volume, Time & Rate of IV Drop*

If you have been provided with a given liquid amount and a period of time, as well as some drop factor in terms of gtts/mL, find out the rate of IV flow required in terms of gtts/min.

Ordinarily, the answer found is rounded either upwards or downwards so that you will be dealing with whole numbers, as it is not feasible for a patient to receive IV in fractions of drops.

The formula you need to use is:

Volume in ml / time in minutes x Drop Factor in gtts/ml

The answer you get using the above formula gives you the rate of IV flow in gtts/min.

### *Illustration: Calculation of IV Flow Rate Given Drop factor & Time*

Find out the rate of IV flow when you need to infuse 1,200ml NS within 6hrs. The drop factor as per the calibration on the infusion set is 15gtts/mL.

The first step in calculating the rate of IV flow is to convert hours into minutes. In this case to convert 6hrs into minutes all you need is multiply 6hrs x 60. The correct answer is 360 minutes.

Now using the formula already highlighted, the workings will be as follows.

1,200ml/360min x 15 gtts/mL

You can begin by dividing 1200 by 360, and using 120 as the divisor 360 will give you 3 while 1,200 will give you 10. At this point your calculations will look like this:

10ml/3min x 15 gtts/mL

You can now cancel out the denominator, where 3min divided by 3 will be 1min and 15gtts/ml divided by 3 will be 5gtts/mL. What remains now is:

10ml/1min x 5gtts/mL or basically: 10ml/1min x 5gtts/1ml

When you calculate 10ml/1min x 5gtts/1ml, the mL units cancel out completely, and what remains from 10mL and 1mL is 10 and 1. So now you have:

10/1min x 5gtts/1, which you can solve by multiplying across

10 x 5gtts = 50gtts and 1min x 1 = 1min.

Your solution is, therefore: 50gtts/1min, which you can simply term 50gtts/min.

### *Illustration: Calculation of IV Flow Rate given Drug & Drop Factor*

Find out the rate of IV flow when the medication record indicates you are to infuse 200mL of 0.9%NaCl IV within a period of 120min and the drop factor is 20gtts/mL.

The formula for IV flow rate remains the same:

Volume in mL/Time in min x Drop Factor in gtts/mL

Substituting for the values provided in the question, you will get:

200ml/120min x 20gtts/mL

You can begin by dividing diagonally using the divisor, 20, so that you end up with 1gtts/mL and 6min as the denominator. Your result so far will look like this:

200ml/6min x 1gtts/mL or 200ml/6min x 1gtts/1ml

The mL units will cancel out completely and you will remain with:

200/6min x 1gtts/1, which when you multiply across gives you: 200gtts/6min

Whereas this answer is correct as a rate, it needs to be simplified further to 33.33gtts/1min or simply 33.33gtts/min. Since the nurse cannot work with fractions where the rate of drop is concerned, the correct acceptable answer is 33.33gtts/min.

## Calculations Involving Maintenance of Fluid

When the medical record has provided the child's weight, it is possible to calculate the quantity of fluid the child requires per day. It is also good to note that hospitals have the leeway to establish their own policies regarding the fluids provided to infants and other children. All the same, it is important for all nurses and other personnel involved in taking care of the young ones to know the basic requirements and how to make the necessary calculations for pediatric dosages and those of adults. Here below are some guidelines commonly in use.

(1) For children whose weight ranges from below 1 kilogram to 10 kilograms, their daily fluid requirement is 100 milliliters per kilogram.

(2) For the children whose weight falls in the range of 10kg to 20kg, their daily fluid requirement is generally 1,000 milliliters, and an additional 50 milliliters for every kilogram of weight above 10 kilograms.

(3) For people whose weight falls in the range of 20 kilograms to 70 kilograms, the daily fluid requirement is generally, 1,500 milliliters, and then 20 milliliters for every kilogram of weight above 20 kilogram.

(4) For people whose weight is above 70 kilograms, the fluid requirement for each person is 2,500 milliliters. This is actually the fluid requirement for adults.

## Illustration: Calculation of Infant's Fluid Requirement Given Weight

When you have an infant whose weight is four kilograms, what would you say the infant's fluid requirement in a day is in terms of milliliters?

Before you proceed with your calculations, you need to establish the infant's age range with regard to fluid requirement. For the infant weight four kilograms, the relevant age range is from below 1 to 10 kilograms. Children whose weight is within this range require 100 milliliters of fluid per kilogram.

You will, therefore, need to multiply 4kg by 100mL per kg, which you can present as:

100ml/1kg x 4kg

The denominator, 1kg, cancels out completely while across only the unit, kg, cancels out. What you are left with is 100mL x 4, which is 400mL.

An infant weight 4kg will, therefore, need 400mL of fluid in a day.

### Illustration: Calculation of Infant's Best IV Flow Rate

There is an infant whose weight is 30.8lbs and you are required to calculate the rate of IV flow in terms of mL per hr if you are to manage to maintain the infant's required level of fluid.

First of all, you need to convert the units that are in lbs to kg, and to do this you simply divide the value you have by 2.2.

30.8lbs divided by 2.2 gives 14 kilograms.

Next, you need to establish the weight range within which the child's weight falls for purposes of fluid infusion. This range is 10kg to 20kg, and the fluid requirement for children whose weight falls within the range is 1,000 milliliters outright, and then an additional 50 milliliters for every additional kilogram of weight coming above 10kg.

So, for this child you need to set aside 1,000ml first for the first 10kg.

Then for the additional 4kg, the calculation should be 50ml x 4, which is 200mL.

When you add the first 1,000mL to the next 200mL, you get 1,200mL, which is the fluid requirement per day for the child weighing 14kg.

### Illustration: Calculating Appropriate Fluid Flow Rate Given Volume & Time

What is the flow rate required if the volume of fluid to be infused is 1,200mL and the period over which it will be given is one day?

To calculate the rate of flow required for this fluid, the formula you need to use is is:

$$\frac{Volume\ of\ fluid}{Period\ of\ time} = \text{Rate of fluid flow in milliliters per hour}$$

Note that the volume in this problem is given in mL, the same unit the formula uses, but the period over which the fluid will be given is given in days yet the formula requires that you give the time element in hours. So, you need to convert the one day given into hours and hence work with 24 hours.

1,200ml/24hr= Rate of fluid flow

The only like terms here are the numbers, and when you divide 1,200 by 24 you get 50. There is 50mL as the numerator and 1 hour or just hr as the denominator, and that constitutes the rate of fluid flow.

In short, the fluid flow rate given the information in the medication record is 50mL/hr.

## Calculations Involving Weight Based Dosage

Sometimes you are provided with the patient's weight and then the dosage is given in weight terms, and you are called upon to find out the dosage to give the patient through your own calculations. Often questions like these involve children, so nurses in the pediatric unit are likely to work with medication records presenting Doctors' orders in this form.

### Dosage Formula Given Weight

With the patient's weight available as well as the required dosage per kilogram, the appropriate dosage to give the patient is calculated using the formula:

Patient's weight in kilograms/recommended dosage per kilogram= Patient's Dosage

### Illustration to Determine if Dr's Dosage is Within Suitable Range

According to the medication record provided by the doctor, a child weighing 15.4lb is to be given 200 milligrams of the drug, Rocephin, and this should be done in 8hr intervals.

According the drug's label, the dosage range under which the dosage of such a child falls is 75 milligrams per kilogram per day to 150 milligrams per kilogram per day or 75mg/kg – 150mg/kg per day. Would you say the medication order given by the doctor fits within the appropriate range?

The way to go about this is to apply the formula suitable for calculating the dosage required, which is:

Weight in Kilograms x Dosage per Kilogram

You notice the child's weight has been provided in lbs, yet the dosage is normally calculated based on kilograms. So it is important to convert the pounds to kilograms.

As stated earlier on, to convert pounds to kilograms you need to divide by 2.2. In this case, 15.4 pounds ÷ 2.2 = 7 kilograms or 7kg.

The minimum dosage for a child who weighs 7kg based on the formula, Weight in Kilograms x Dosage per Kilogram, is:

7 kilograms x 75 milligrams per Kilogram

The answer for this is 525 milligrams, meaning the least you can administer to this child and be doing the right thing is 525mg.

Next you need to calculate the upper limit, the maximum amount of the drug you can administer to this child without risking the child's health.

The formula remains the same and what changes is only the amount of drug per kilogram. In this case it is 150mg/kg. So, based on Weight in Kilograms x Dosage per Kilogram:

7 kilograms x 150 milligrams per kilogram = 1,050mg

You now need to determine the amount to administer each time with 8hrs in between. Begin by dividing a day by 8hrs, and the best way to do this is to convert a day into hours so that you now have 24hrs ÷ 8hrs, which gives 3.

If you go by the medication order given by the doctor, you would administer 200mg three times a day, which is 200mg x 3 = 600mg.

Remember you have established the safe range for the medication to be 525 milligrams to 1,050 milligrams. Obviously, the 600mg per day the doctor prescribed falls within that range of 525mg – 1,050mg. So, as for the question, would you say the medication order given by the doctor fits within the appropriate range the answer is, certainly, yes.

### *Illustration on Calculation of Dosage in mL*

The doctor orders the drug, Solumedrol, 1.5mg/kg for a patient who weighs 74.8lb. The drug at the hospital has dosage provided in 125mg/2mL. The question you need to answer through the necessary calculations is the number of milliliters the nurse needs to administer.

Using the formula: Weight in Kilograms x Dosage per Kilogram, your calculation should follow the steps shown below, but first the patient's weight needs to be converted to kilograms.

To convert 74.8lb to kilograms, all you need to do is calculate 74.8lb ÷ 2.2, which gives 34kg. Since the doctor has ordered 1.5mg/kg, this translates to:

1.5mg x 34kg for the patient, which is, 51mg

The next point to consider is that the drug at the nurse' disposal has dosage given in terms of mg/mL, essentially, 125mg/2mL. How do you establish the amount of drug in milliliters to administer to the patient? The correct formula, as has been stated earlier on, is:

Amount ordered / amount in dosage available x Volume per Rate Available = Required amount of liquid

For this specific question, your calculations would be:

51mg/125mg x 2mL

Right away the mg units above and below will cancel out. Then when you calculate 51 ÷ 125 you get 0.408

Now you can calculate 0.408 x 2mL, and the result will be 0.816mL, which you can round off to 2 decimal places to have 0.82mL. So to answer the question asked, the nurse needs to administer 0.82mL of the available drug.

### Calculations Involving Mass over Time & IV Rate

When a doctor issues an order and gives it in mass quantity over a given period of time, you may be required to calculate the appropriate rate of IV flow in terms of milliliters per hour based on the mass per volume provided. You will often find these kinds of calculations where members of medical staff are providing critical nursing care.

The appropriate formula for such a case is:

Amount ordered per hour / amount available x Volume in mL = Rate of IV flow in mL per hr

### Illustration on Calculation of Infusion Flow Rate in mL/hr

Administer to the patient the drug, Dopamine, 500mg in 250mL within D5W, and carry out the infusion at the rate of 20 milligrams per hour. Now you need to calculate the rate of infusion flow in milliliters per hour.

The appropriate formula to use is:

Amount ordered per hour / amount available x Volume in milliliters = Rate of IV flow in milliliters per hour

In this case, your calculation should look as shown below.

20mg per hr/500mg x 250mL

The easiest move to begin with would be to divide 250 and 500 with the common divisor, 250, and you would remain with:

20mg per hour/2mg x 1mL

The mg units above and below can now cancel out, and when you multiply across, 20 per how x 1mL, you would have 20mL per hour. But then you have the denominator 2, and 20ml per hour/2 = 10mL per hr or 10mL/hr.

In short, the required rate of infusion flow in terms of mL per hr is 10mL/hr.

### Illustration on Calculation of Infusion Pump Flow Rate

A doctor prescribes the drug, Aggrastat, for a patient whose weight is 100 kilograms. The dosage as per the medication record is 12.5mg in a liquid 250mL, and the nurse concerned is to infuse the medication at the rate of 6 micrograms or mcg per kilogram or kg per hour/hr. What is the flow rate appropriate for setting the pump at in milliliters per hour or mL/hr?

To calculate the appropriate rate of flow, you need to use the formula:

Amount ordered per hour / amount available x Volume in milliliters or mL = Appropriate Rate of Flow in mL/hr

Begin by converting the amount ordered per hour into the amount appropriate for the patient. Considering this question falls under the category of dosage provided as per the patient's weight, you need to use the patient's 100kg as well as the dosage rate of 6mcg per kg per hr.

The patient's right dosage = Patient's Weight in Kg x Dosage given in Kg

Patient's Weight in Kg x Dosage given in Kg = The patient's right dosage

100 kilograms x 6 micrograms per kg per hour = 600mcg per hr (right dosage)

You now need to convert the 600mcg per hour to mg per hour. The formula alredy provided for this is dividing by 1,000.

600mcg ÷ 1,000 = 0.6mg per hr(mg/hr)

Now you have the units needed to calculate the flow rate of the infusion pump. This is how you do the calculation:

0.6mg per hour / 12.5mg x 250mL

If you begin by canceling 12.5 against 250, 12.5 divided by 12.5 gives 1 while 250 divided by 12.5 gives 20. You now have:

0.6mg per hour/1mg x 20mL

The mg units can cancel out completely above and below, and you can now multiply the units across.

0.6 per hr x 20mL = 12 milliliters per hour or mL/hr

# Chapter 9: Math and the Nursing Career

You may wish to be a nurse but have no idea if nursing has categories, and if that is the case you will benefit a lot from this chapter. After taking the basic nursing course, you could choose to specialize by training or by gaining relevant experience in an area you prefer. However, it is important to note that no single area of nursing will shield you from basic math and dosing calculations. Even for those nurses who are engaged to take care of individual invalids, they deal with math when counting the medications taken and medications remaining. Moreover, they are in a position to question any prescription issued to a patient where the dosage looks unreasonable. They also understand what constitutes overdosing, including dispensing medications within unduly close intervals.

Still, do not hasten to get into nursing without a clear picture of what you would want to major in. Take some time and learn about the nursing industry and all the nursing careers that are available in the market. Remember, you can even specialize in more than one field of nursing. For example, you can be a pediatric nurse and still be an ER nurse.

### *Why there is Great Potential in the Nursing Career*

In a few years time, nurses will be in high demand because the older generation is still aging and so are the nurses from this generation. This means that the older generation of nurses will soon retire and they will give way to the younger generation of nurses. Statistics show that by the year 2020, there is going to be about 1.7 million job vacancies in the nursing field.

There has been a steady rise in demand of nurses over the past few decades and this continues to be the case today. As such, the nursing career is still growing unlike many other careers and sectors of the economy. Statistics show that between 1981 and 2009, there was an astounding rise in the population of people who were enrolling into nursing courses and the numbers have continued to rise. For you to have a competitive advantage over other nursing students, it is recommended that you pursue an advanced degree that will earn you a higher salary and greater benefits.

### The Certified Nursing Assistant

The role of a CNA is to offer support to patients under an LPN or RN supervisor. As a CNA, you are not limited in terms of work environment so you may work in any medical setting, from the ER to a home care setting. You can acquire a CNA certification from a local community based college that offers the course and once you have gained your certification, you can now assess whether you would want a job in the capacity of an RN or not. You can also use your experience as a CNA to apply for ADN programs.

### The Invaluable School Nurse

For you to qualify for a school nurse position, you should have baccalaureate degree or RN certificate. A School nurse plays a vital role in taking care of student's health in school. As a school nurse, your main job is to provide therapeutic care to students when they fall ill in class, give first aid as needed and administer prescribed medication as indicated by a consulted physician. You are also allowed to administer medication for mild illness such as flu and stomach ache. As a school nurse you are likely to get lower salaries than other nurses in your field, however, you get to enjoy long holidays and summer breaks during which you can advance your nursing studies or volunteer in other health facilities.

### Nurses Specializing in Handling HIV/AIDS

The HIV care nurses offer both medical and emotional support to patients living with the virus. For you to become a HIV/AIDS nurse, you need to have an ADN and RN license but it is also an added advantage when you have had some experience handling HIV/AIDS patients. Apart from administering medication to your patients and assisting the doctor, it is important to build a friendly nurse-patient relationship with your patients and offer moral support as much as possible. As a way of giving back to the community, you can use your free time to educate the community on how the disease is spread, how to prevent it and how to handle and care for people in the community who are living with HIV/AIDS.

### The Radiology Nurse

For you to become a radiology care giver you are required to have a BSN or ADN certification and no former experience is necessary. The main role of a radiology nurse is to prepare a patient for a procedure. Some patients come in for MRIs, ultrasounds, CT scans and other tests and you are expected to prepare them both physically and mentally for the procedure. Because a patient only comes in for the procedure and leaves, there is no opportunity to create a patient-nurse relationship.

## Nurses within the American Red Cross

To work with Red Cross as a nurse you need to have at least an RN license, BSN or ADN. Nurses who work with Red Cross also have an opportunity to go through CNA training course. As a Red Cross nurse you get to travel all around the country and in some cases, all over the world providing emergency care. Your duties include providing medical care, providing disaster relief as well as support for needy patients.

## The Public Health Nurse

Typically, all you need to be a public health nurse is RN license or a BSN degree. A health nurse can easily get employment through a local municipality or county. The main responsibilities you will have as a public health caregiver is providing education to the entire community, creating vaccination programs, and running surveys to identify risk factors of different types of ailments. It is also your duty to identify certain conditions such as bad roads that need improvement so that the community can have access to health care.

## Nurses Specialized in Nutrition and Fitness

Nurses who would want to specialize in fitness and nutrition should be licensed RNs and have an ADN or a diploma that is equivalent to that. As a fitness and nutrition nurse your main responsibility is to offer support and nutrition advice to patients who require exercise and proper diet to manage their lives. The advantage of being a fitness and nutrition nurse is that you are not limited to the environment where you can offer your services. You may work in a spa, medical clinic, gym, hospital and any medical clinics.

## The Oncology Nurse

With an RN certification and a BSN degree, you can comfortably make a living as an oncology nurse. Most oncology nurses earn an average salary of up to $70,000 but this can vary depending on what medical facility you are in. As an oncology nurse, your main duty is to care for patients with cancer and those at a high risk of getting cancer. You can work in a clinic, hospital or even a private medical setting. You are also required to monitor every patient personally and administer medication to the patients as prescribed. It is important to build a friendly nurse-patient relationship with your patients and encourage them in every way possible.

## Nurses Specialized in Neonatal Intensive Care Unit

A NICU nurse is situated in a Neonatal Intensive care Unit in local hospitals. For you to become a NICU nurse, you must hold a BSN as well as a RN certificate. After becoming a NICU nurse, you can also decide to join an MSN program and graduate to a neonatal nurse practitioner. It is also advisable for a NICU nurse to spend some quality time in clinical training so that you can be fully prepared for the responsibilities that come with this career. As a NICU care giver, you are responsible for sick newborns and premature babies.

The kind of care that these newborns need is very demanding and not everyone can handle this kind of work environment. That said, you need to be sure that you can handle babies in such a delicate stage before pursuing such a career. Some of the newborns under your care will require surgery, some need ventilators to breathe while some require to remain in incubators and it your responsibility to ensure that each one gets the care that they need. You may need to also provide emotion support to the parents and families of these babies as they try to come into terms with the condition of their babies.

### Nurse Handling Plastic Surgery

With a BSN or ADN, you can become a plastic surgery nurse. However, a BSN is often preferred over an AND because a nurse with a BSN can assist in complex procedures like a craniofacial reconstructive procedure. Your main role as a plastic surgery nurse is to provide the care needed for patients who are about to undergo medically compulsory procedures or elective procedures. You can also offer emotional support to patients with congenital conditions or facial deformities. In some clinics, a nurse also acts as an assistant helping in face peeling procedures and liposuction.

### Nurses working within Prisons & Other Correction Facilities

For this kind of nursing, you are mostly required to have an MSN or BSN degree as well as a RN license. A prison nurse is basically supposed to look after the health of inmates. This is a career that requires an objective and strong willed mind because it is easy to handle a patient as one who committed certain crimes rather than one who needs medical attention.

As a prison nurse, you should give first aid and all the necessary care to inmates who are injured while in incarceration, administer treatment to both acute and chronic illnesses as well as ensure that every inmate is in a good health condition.

### Nurses Charged with Rehabilitation

For you to work as a rehabilitation nurse, you need to have a BSN as well as a RN license. In this kind of work, it is important to have a good relationship with your patient because most of the care that you will need to give is in the form of emotional support and encouragement. There is a lot of emotional responsibility that comes with this kind of nursing because some patients are in denial or are in a difficult stage of recovery as they try to adapt to their new lifestyle and so they need all the support they can get.

A rehabilitation nurse mostly deals with patients who have had life altering accidents, chronic illnesses or patients with disabilities. As a rehabilitation nurse, you are required to administer medication and perform physiotherapy. In some cases you are required to also help a patient re-learn how to move and walk again as you also teach some skills all over again for those patients who have lost their capability.

### Nurses Handling Labor & Delivery

To be a delivery nurse you must be RN certified and hold a BSN or ADN degree. As a delivery nurse, you have the privilege of bringing life into the world. A delivery nurse is supposed to give moral support to a mother in the delivery room, monitor the condition of the mother and the baby during the entire labor process and provide the support needed by both of them after delivery. You are also required to help the moms in their recovery process from labor and where necessary hold the baby up when the mother is breastfeeding. Sometimes moms may need to rest and so it is your duty to take the babies away into the nursery for a period of time.

### Nurses Handling Burns

This is a demanding profession and one that is not for the faint hearted. For you to qualify for this career, you should hold a masters in a related field of medicine. When you are a burn care nurse, you deal with all kinds of burns on patients from burns caused by chemicals, fires, hot liquids and many others. You are required to give pain medication to patients who are in pain, provide skin and wound care and also give moral and emotional support to patients in their recovery journey. You are also supposed to educate families and persons who handle the patients so that they are able to take care of them both emotionally and physically.

### The Invaluable Surgical Nurses

For you to become a surgical nurse, you are required to go through a peri-operative nurse program, hold a RN license as well as a BSN. The main role of a surgical nurse is to help the surgeon in an operating room. Before any procedure, you should get the operating room ready and ensure that all equipment is sterile. During a procedure, you may also be required to provide some form of support to a conscious patient. There are various types of nurses in the surgical field such as scrub nurses, a circulating nurse and first assistant.

### Nurses for Pediatric Home Care

If you want to be a pediatric home care nurse, then you need a BSN or ADN degree as well as a RN certificate. As a homecare pediatric nurse, you get to offer a range of medical services to your patients in their homes. You can provide care to a new born who has added care needs as well as other older children in the family who have different medical conditions. It is also your responsibility to advice parents on the way to care for and handle their needy children. You should also monitor the child's progress when you are both near and away.

### The Forensic Nurse

With an eye for detail, a BSN degree and RN certification, you can get into forensic nursing which is a career that involves legal professionals and law enforcement that help to investigate crimes. A forensic nurse helps victims of crimes such as rape, domestic violence and robbery to recover both medically and emotionally. As you help your patients, it is easy for you as a forensic nurse to become traumatized because of all the crime scenes you are exposed to and the disturbing conditions that you witness your patients in and so it is important for you to regularly go for therapy.

### The Geriatric Nurse

A geriatric nurse looks after senior patients in hospitals, assisted living homes, clinic settings and other forms of health facilities. For you to become a geriatric nurse, you need to be a BSN degree holder. Among the duties you are required to handle are administering medication, walking the patients, feeding them and also offering support to the patient's family. For those patients who are likely to develop conditions such as cancer, dementia and Alzheimer's disease, you are required to focus on how to offer preventative care.

### Nurses Providing Care in Rural Settings

A rural caregiver serves in marginalized communities or those that do not have any access to proper hospital services. You can offer to travel to your patients especially if they lack access to public transportation that can get them to your services. A rural caregiver can also educate the community on issues such as safe medical practices, hygiene practices and diseases prevention. For you to qualify as a rural nurse, you should have either a BSN or ADN degree and also be RN certified.

### The ER Nurse

An ER nurse should be RN certified and hold a BSN or ADN degree from a recognized institution. The responsibilities of ER nurses depend on what kind of care an ER is authorized to give in a specific hospital. Some hospitals will allow you to only provide basic first aid care for emergencies while some hospitals expect you as an ER nurse to provide trauma care services for serious emergencies such as injuries caused by gunshots and car crashes. You may also perform minor procedures, prepare patients to be admitted or discharged from hospital, administer medicine as well as monitor a patient's health condition.

### Nurses Providing Long-Term Care

For you to become a certified long-term care nurse, you need to have an RN license, a BSN or CDN degree and a CPR certification that is current. CNAs offering long-term nursing care can pursue RN licensing degree and secure a career in long-term nursing. As a long-term care giver you can work in several settings such as residential homes that care for needy adults, nursing homes and any kind of medical facilities. Other than the basic health care, you may also be required to provide assistance such as walking a patient, bathing them and performing other tasks that they are not in a position to perform alone.

### Nurses of the Intensive Care Unit

If you decide that you want to be an ICU nurse, you must attain an ADN degree and become RN licensed. In some hospitals, they give preference to nurses with a BSN degree and several years of experience as a nurse in any hospital setting. As an ICU nurse, you are required to be alert and quick to respond to any emergencies because most of the patients in the ICU are in life-threatening conditions that can fluctuate any time. These are often people who have gone through invasive surgery, traumatic injury and or life threatening illness and so they should be handled in a delicate manner.

### The Pediatric Nurse

A holder of an ASN degree qualifies to be a pediatric nurse but having a BSN degree is even more sort after in the market. A nurse who holds a BSN is often paid higher than one who only has an ASN degree. As a pediatric nurse, you can choose to work in any medical setting such as clinics, children hospitals, pediatrician offices and many other settings. If you love being around children, then this is a fulfilling career for you as you get to treat and spend time with children. Depending on the work setting, a pediatric can administer vaccination, treat minor cuts and wounds, offer supportive care, extract foreign objects and carry out many other tasks.

### The Hospice Care Nurse

The minimum requirement needed for you to become a hospice care giver is mostly an LPN certification. An RN license and a BSN certification is also an added advantage in the job market for hospice care givers. In fact, hospice care givers with a BSN certification are paid higher than those with an LPN certification. An intake nurse ensures that there is a smooth transition for the patient from the hospital setting to a hospice care setting.

You can provide care in either a home-care setting or a hospice home. Your main role as a hospice care giver is to offer palliative care to the patient, administer pain drugs and assist in day to day activities that the patient cannot perform on their own. You are also supposed to provide emotional support to both the patient and his or her family. The patient's family needs to be prepared mentally for loss and grief and it is part of your duty to ensure that they are emotionally prepared.

### Nurses Handling Telephonic Triage

These are nurses who provide their services over the telephone. For you to be a telephonic triage nurse, you need to be a sharp listener and quick in giving solutions. When a patient is not able to access a doctor's office, you as a telephonic triage nurse can listen to a patient's symptoms via the telephone and advice them appropriately on the right course of action. You can work for a hospital, insurance company or any medical facility that requires such services.

### Opportunities of a Nurse Educator

For you to be a qualified nurse educator you need to get an RN license and also complete an MSN at the very least. Some universities and colleges also require that you get a DPN. Your main role as a nurse educator is to teach and educate students as you prepare them for their nursing career. You can still decide to further your education as a nurse educator by enrolling in research and clinical programs that can help you keep up with the latest developments in medicine.

### Opportunities for an Epidemics Research Nurse

If you have a keen eye and a passion for research, then this is the nursing career for you. Your work as an epidemic research nurse is to carry out research on epidemics so as to find solutions and prevention plans that can be applied. A research nurse often works in a laboratory or clinical setting alongside fellow scientists and doctors. Research nurses are able to observe a patient who has contracted an illness that has epidemic potential and provide possible solutions to the epidemic. For you to become a certified research nurse, you need to have an RN license as well as a BSN degree. An DNP and MSN degree is also an added advantage.

### Opportunities for a Dialysis Nurse

A dialysis nurse cares for patients with kidney failure who often times are also diabetic. As a dialysis care giver, some of the responsibilities you have are to prepare a patient for the dialysis procedure, offer support throughout the entire dialysis process and advice the patient on how to manage their condition. You can work in both outpatient dialysis medical clinics and in hospitals as long as you have the qualifications needed to be a dialysis nurse. For you to be certified, you should have an RN license and hold a BSN. You can however also work in the capacity of renal dialysis care givers with a diploma or ADN certification.

### Opportunities for a Bioterrorism Nurse

For you to qualify as a bioterrorism caregiver, you need to have an RN license as well as critical care and emergency room experience. This is a field that requires you to have speed and the ability to function under pressure or chaos. The role of a bioterrorism nurse is similar to that of a disaster nurse in the sense that they all care for casualties during a tragedy. As a bioterrorism nurse however, you are required to seek out casualties during other crisis such as war and terrorism.

### Important Role of Senior Home Care Nurse

As a senior care nurse, your duty is to take care of senior patients in health care facilities, a nursing home or in an assisted living community. The responsibilities of a senior home care nurse are mainly like those of a geriatric nurse but because services are rendered in the senior patient's residency, you may be required to help with other daily activities such as bathing, caring for wounds especially for patients with diabetes, dressing, and giving medication.  If you would like to get into this career, then you should take up a two to three year degree course in nursing to become a registered home care nurse.

### Opportunities for Legal Nurse Consultant

You need an RN licensing, a degree in BSN as well as a few years of nursing experience to qualify as a nurse consultant. Your duties as a legal nurse consultant include collecting relevant documentation needed to prepare a court case, providing reliable testimony in front of a jury or judge, providing support to attorneys on any side of the case and acting as an advisor in cases dealing with worker's compensation, medical malpractice, personal injury and insurance fraud cases.

### *Opportunities for the Pharmaceutical Research Nurse*

Should you decide that this is the profession you want to be in, you can take up a course in any recognized university that offers certificate in the clinical research department for nurses in pharmaceutical research. With a BSN or MSN degree, you can also apply for this kind of profession. As a pharmaceutical nurse, you can work in universities or a pharmaceutical company to monitor certain clinical tests, assist in enrolling patients for clinical trials and also providing advice and guidance on medical strategies.

### *Interesting Opportunities for the Flight Transport Nurse*

As a flight transport nurse, your role is to accompany a patient as they are air lifted to a medical facility. You are expected to monitor as well as give medical support to the patient right from the ground and you can also assist in transferring the patient from the ambulance to the plane. You can land a job in a private hospital or in emergency facilities that offer air lifting services. Some affluent society members also employ flight transport nurses who can be called upon when there is an emergency.

### *Opportunities for the Occupational Health Nurse*

You can find employment as an occupational health nurse mostly in plants, factories, ongoing building sites, fire stations and any other place where risk of getting injured in the line of duty is high. Your role is to mainly treat injuries and illnesses that occur at the workplace and to maintain a safe working environment for all those who work in the area.

### *Adventures of a Cruise Ship Nurse*

If you would like to travel around the world and still care for patients then this is the job for you. As a ship nurse, your sole responsibility is to treat acute illnesses and give first aid to passengers or staff aboard the ship. A common illness that a cruise ship nurse has to deal with is passengers who get sea sick and when providing such care it may mean that you will work each day of the voyage. For you to become a cruise ship nurse, you need to get a CPR certification, an ACLS certification, be a holder of a BSN degree and have at least two years working experience in a critical care facility or an emergency setting.

### *Management Role of the* **Charge Nurse**

With an MSN or BSN degree, you are qualified to be a charge nurse. Your main role as a charge nurse is to ensure that your unit is well managed and that all patients receive the best care that is available to them. Your work is similar to that of an administrative nurse because your responsibilities involve scheduling and managing your unit. As a charge nurse, you may work independently in your unit or under supervision by the overall charge nurse.

### Opportunities for the Wound Ostomy Continence Nurse

A wound ostomy nurse cares for patients who have healing incisions, wounds and patients who have ostomies. Your main role is to administer medication, provide pain relief options, treat wounds and help the patients know how they should care for the condition in their homes. For you to give this specialized care, you should be RN licensed, have a BSN degree or higher, go through a WOCN-approved course and have relevant clinical exposure.

### Opportunities for Nursing in Infusion Therapy

For you to become this type of a care giver, you need to have either a BSN or ADN degree from a recognized program as well as RN licensing. Your main role is to administer IV medication, insert any IV lines for the patient as needed as well as provide any other needed support to the patient. You are not limited to where you can work since you can be employed in a clinic, hospital, in a home or any type of medical facility.

### Role of the Coordinating Transplant Nurse

A transplant nurse coordinator works with patients who need organ transplants. You can help in determining whether a patient needs an organ transplant or not, seek out a possible match for the organ and inform the patient when there is an organ available. You can also help in assessing if a patient is eligible for an organ transplant, for example, an alcoholic who still struggles with alcoholism may not be a suitable recipient of another liver. For you to become a transplant nurse coordinator, you need to have a BSN and RN licensing.

### Nursing Opportunities in Psychiatric Mental Health

For you to become a certified psychiatric mental health nurse, you need to be RN licensed and hold a BSN degree. If you wish to become an advanced psychiatric health nurse (PMH-APRNs) you can enroll in a master's program. Your main role as a psychiatric health nurse is to care for patients with mental health problems in hospitals, mental health institutions and homes. You are required to give medication, plan and implement care plans and care for any other needs they may have. You can also help in diagnosing other health conditions that your patients have.

### How to Practice as a Family Nurse

As a family nurse practitioner, you will mostly work in medical practices or clinics. Your main role is to offer diagnostic care, give treatment options and prescribe medication. In communities where there are no medical facilities, a family caregiver can also provide the primary care needed in that community. For you to be a family caregiver practitioner you need to have a master's or an advanced doctorate degree.

### Opportunities for Nursing in the Medical-Surgical Practice

For you to become a medical-surgical practitioner you will need to have a master's degree and pass the board certification for medical-surgical nurses. As a surgical nurse your role in the operating room is very vital before and after an operation. You are required to give before and after operative support and care to patients, assist in preparing anesthesia and prepare the patient both physically and mentally before the procedure.

### Nursing Opportunities in the Control of Infectious Diseases

Your main role as an infectious control nurse is to prevent infectious diseases from spreading. You are required to quarantine patients as well as contain areas that have been affected by an infectious disease to avoid more cases of infection and educate or sensitize the people of that given area. With such a career you are most likely to work with a government agency, hospitals and other health facilities. For you to be certified as an infectious disease control nurse, you are required to have RN licensing as well as a MSN degree but you can also sit for the AIPC examination.

### Nursing Opportunities in Health Administration

These nurses have supervisory roles to play in nursing homes, laboratories and hospitals. As a health administration nurse, your duty is to come up with operating budgets to be used by your nursing staff, creating schedules and overseeing the overall patient's care. Having a BSN degree is the most important qualification you are required to have in this career but having an MSN degree is also an added advantage.

### Nursing Role in Disaster Management

Your main role as a management nurse is to deal with several aspects of disaster management, prevention and care. You are responsible for working with the local municipality to come up with a disaster prevention and management plan and provide response to disaster emergencies. When there is a disaster, you can give first aid, perform triage and give emotional support to victims of the disaster. For you to qualify as a disaster management nurse you need RN licensing as well as a BSN but some employers ask for an MSN as well.

### *Interesting Role as a Travel Nurse*

A travel nurse may provide RN services or work in several specialty practices. Your main role as a travel nurse is to work in hand with an employment agency in order to fill positions in health facilities that need to be filled or that are understaffed. If you like to travel and do not mind living in different places all the time then this is a perfect job for you because you will be required to move from city to city for certain periods. The pay is often high because there is a high demand for care givers all over. All you need to qualify as a traveling nurse is RN licensing and a BSN or ADN degree.

### *Role of a Nursing Practitioner*

As a nurse practitioner, you are required to provide essential services that are beyond what a typical nurse provides. You can diagnose an ailment, see patients and prescribe medication pretty much as a doctor should. When there is a shortage of doctors, nurse practitioners can fill up these gaps. You can either work in hospital settings or urgent care facilities. For you to qualify as a practitioner, you must have a master's degree.

### *Role of the Nursing* **Anesthetist**

As an anesthetics nurse, you are required to work with an anesthesiologist or other physicians in operation rooms. Your main role is to administer anesthesia and monitor the patient's vital signs. You have to have sharp math and deduction skills because you need to make calculations for anesthesia doses and also administer medication to the patient in the correct way. You must be certified through NBCR and have a graduate degree for you to qualify as an anesthetist nurse.

### *Role of the Certified Nurse Midwife*

Certified nurse mid-wives play an important role especially to patients who are not in a position to get to a medical facility. Your main role as a nurse midwife is to offer parental care, postpartum care as well as family planning services. All you need to be a certified nurse midwife is a CNM certificate and a BSN.

### *Role of the Neonatal Nurse Practitioner*

These nurses work in the NICU with fellow NICU nurses. You work as a neonatal nurse is to take care of premature babies with medical complications. Typically, neonatal nurses are situated in level 2 and 3 units where there are more serious cases. For you to qualify as a NNP, you need to have RN licensing, neonatal resuscitation certificate as well as a master's degree.

# Chapter 9: Dosing Math for the Pharmacist

There is a lot of math in pharmacy although it may appear to the layman as if the role of pharmacists, and even pharmacy technicians, is solely to hand over medications to customers or patients. Actually, like other medics, pharmacists and their staff take their major goal as that of improving health for the public, as they ensure medications are properly dispensed and utilized for effective outcome.

In pursuing this goal, pharmacists and fellow technicians seek to attain as well as maintain expansive knowledge as well as skills. Anyone who has attempted the exams set for Pharmacy Technicians can attest to how solid it is, with a good part of it comprising questions targeting entry of medication orders as well as the process of filling up prescriptions. Candidates are tested on their capacity to calculate medication doses, and how well they are able to covert values in a given unit of measure to equivalent values in a different unit. This essentially means that math is inevitable when it comes to working in the field of pharmacy.

In fact, math is central in the success of a person trying to advance their career as pharmacist. It is also extremely important in ensuring the safety of the patients whose outcome depends on the right dispensing of medication doses. In short, math is indispensable when it comes to pharmacy work, and whether it is the pharmacists or the pharmacy technicians involved, they must be competent in math.

When it comes to day to day calculations done within the pharmacy, they involve, among other details, measurement units and calculation methods. No wonder pharmacists are expected to be good at math because there are numerous math based problems to solve before dispensing medication to patients or release drugs to various departments or wards within a health institution. Sometimes members of pharmacy staff are expected to do some dimensional analysis, use ratio and proportions, and even convert units of one kind to another. Sometimes a pharmacist is required to do a series of computations in order to determine the exact amount of drug to be released for the day.

Pharmacists also have to be competent at calculating concentration level of various medicinal preparations and dilutions, as well as determining the appropriate dosing for individual patients. The value equivalents between different units that help pharmacy staff in their computations are the same ones used by medical practitioners who write prescriptions, nurses who dispensed medications as per the medication records, and every other medical staff involved in dispensing medications of different kinds to patients.

## The Role of Clinical Pharmacists in Linking Patients and Physicians

In the past ten years or so, clinical pharmacies have advanced in the kind of professional services they offer and this has earned them a place among the significant players in the health care system. Your main role as a clinical pharmacist is to interact with both the patient and physician and act as a bridge between these two.

Your knowledge on prescriptions and therapeutics as well as your constant interaction with medication prescribers puts you in an ideal place to offer services needed by both patients and doctors. The Association of clinic pharmacists and clinicians provides a base for assured quality care for patients. One of the key features that marked a major milestone in the field of pharmacy was having clinical pharmacists working in the ward. As a clinical pharmacist, you can now participate in taking ward rounds together with a physician and offer recommendations or suggestions to the physician when necessary.

One of your main responsibilities is to check the prescription written by the physician and ensure that it falls within all the prescription rules and recommendations. You are supposed to check whether it is the correct drug and whether all the details such as the dose, time, dosage and duration are indicated correctly. If you notice any inconsistency or error in the prescription, it is your duty to make the appropriate corrections and present the issue to the prescribing physician after which you are supposed to document that intervention. If both you and the physician agree on the corrections made, you are supposed to document it also. Agreeing on the matter also means that your intervention was correct.

As a clinical pharmacist, there are many responsibilities that fall within your docket. You can participate in reviewing medication, identifying medication related issues, giving therapeutic recommendations, promoting medication compliance, obtaining and reviewing medication and medical history of patients to check for medication errors among other responsibilities. What you should mainly look out for when checking for medication errors is dispensing, prescription, and also administration errors. Other responsibilities that fall under your career may include identifying drug interactions, counseling patients, monitoring adverse medication reactions, advising on how to use medication and some medical devices such as insulin pens, inhalers, nasal sprays and eye drops. Your participation in ICU or ward rounds as well as clinical discussions can play a big role in identifying, preventing or reducing drug interactions.

Additionally, you can play a part in developing patient compliant programs that are cost effective and also help in creating databases for every drug and every clinic trial. Clinical pharmacists have a wealth of knowledge and are always updated on the dynamic world of health and medicine and this can allow you to contribute greatly in clinical research projects as well as ongoing research projects. You are also authorized to carry out drug dilutions, dose calculations and extemporaneous preparations. The services offered in a clinical pharmacy help to develop as well as maintain clinical practices that focus on quality patient care.

### *Importance of Clinical Pharmacists in different Departments*

As a clinical pharmacist, you are supposed to conduct patient interviews to enquire on their medical history, family and social history, use of any OTC drugs, history of any allergy, alternative medication systems and dietary supplements. Performing a drug therapy review aids in recognizing and utilizing the relevant lab and clinic data available to identify as well as resolve issues related to medication such as therapy duplication, drug-food and drug-drug interactions, inappropriate dosage, contraindications, potential ADRs, incorrect medication selection, lack of drug therapy description, non-adherence to drugs and provision of better and cost effective solutions. You can also be part of making therapeutic decisions and preparing guidelines for the use of antibiotics by assessing their cost effectiveness.

Another major responsibility of a clinical pharmacist is providing updated and unbiased data on any area of medication use. You are required to give information regarding the strength, cost, brand and the available drug formulations of certain drugs in the health sector. You are also responsible for providing information on empirical dosages in patients who have impairment of hepatic or renal function. With the vast knowledge you have on medication, you can be able to tell apart original medication and counterfeit medication and this is an important aspect of drug monitoring. A clinical pharmacist can also participate actively in medical camps, therapeutic medication monitoring as well as patient awareness initiatives that educate people on drug use.

As a clinical pharmacist, you should ensure that dilution, reconstitution, storage, stability, compatibility as well as administering of medication are done appropriately. You can also aid in converting paenterals to oral doses when it is indicated. Another major responsibility is providing alert cards to selected patients suffering from adverse drug reactions or those taking drugs which require special caution such as those taking insulin, aspirin, warfarin, drug allergy medications, epilepsy medication and cardiac problems medications.

If you are a clinical pharmacist you can work in a neonatology or pediatric unit, where you are responsible for calculating dosage as well as modifying dosage forms. There is a high demand for clinical pharmacists in the neonatology and pediatric units who can calculate dosages, dilute pediatric medication as well as adjust doses depending on the patient's weight, age, surface area and gestation age. You can also assist in preparing neonatal/pediatric formulary and counseling or educating parents regarding immunization and medication.

If you are working in a stroke unit, you can help in reducing adverse effects caused by drug interactions by identifying and monitoring certain risk groups of people. Some of the patients who may be at risk of getting adverse effects from medication are patients who depend heavily on warfarin. You can advice a doctor on how to adjust a patient's dose in order to manage any potential side effects. You can also counsel a patient on how to manage a proper diet, how to manage adverse effects of medication as well as INR monitoring. When you are working in an oncology department, your main responsibility is to calculate the surface area for a patient who is just about to have a chemotherapy session based on his or her weight and height.

Failing to adjust medication dosage can cause an increase in mortality and morbidity rates and also drive up the cost of therapeutic interventions. A good example of medication dosage that can be adjusted is that of patients who have renal impairments. As a clinical pharmacist, you are required to confirm the list of medication that is ordered prior to delivery. It is recommended that you monitor creatinine clearance before ordering and ensure that the right dosing guidelines are used. You can adjust a dose through dose reduction or interval extension. Renal function estimates will help you to determine which patients need shorter intervals between doses and those that need smaller amount of the dose over a long period of time.

People who have gone through organ transplantation are required to take many drugs for them to avoid graft rejection and recover fully. Part of your duty as a clinical pharmacist in this case is to counsel or educate these patients on how they can modify their lifestyles and use the prescribed medication correctly for them to get full recovery.

There is a great need for clinical pharmacists all over and indeed more medical care givers should consider taking up a course in clinical pharmacy. A study done on the events of adverse drug reactions and medical errors found that more than five hundred thousand cases of adverse drug effects which cost a total of almost $800 were reported. One of the ways we can remedy this situation is by having more clinical pharmacists in the wards as well as other medical health facilities.

Clinical pharmacists can improve medical efficiency in the health facilities by providing invaluable knowledge on dosing and medical use, working closely with patients in improving their adherence to medication requirements, consulting other health care givers on medication-related problems, reviewing patients medical history and determining the right medication interventions for them as well as providing guidance in cases where a patient is on several medication to simplify their medication regimens.

In many instances, clinical pharmacists work hand in hand with their patients doing tasks such as conducting detailed medical reviews on patients, helping to solve medication problems that the patients may face, motivating the patients by helping them adhere to the medication requirements and participating in group meetings with patients to address patient's needs.

Having a clinical pharmacist as a significant member of a primary care giving team increases efficiency in the medical department, relieves some workload off the other care providers and ensures that the team stays updated at all times on the best practices. Clinical pharmacists also enhance the quality of care given by working with the patients so as to improve on medication management, medication adherence and medication safety.

### Hospital Pharmacists vs Clinical Pharmacists

Even though both the hospital and the clinical nurses are concerned with providing medication for their patients, they have a varying scope of responsibilities. The main role of a hospital pharmacist is to prepare medication prescriptions for a patient while that of a clinical pharmacist is to directly interact with the patient on all matters regarding medication. A clinical pharmacist is required to have additional training over and above the type of training that a hospital nurse has. This means that one should have a complete residency and at least one professional degree. That inevitably means that clinic nurses are paid higher salaries than their counterparts.

Both pharmacists are expected to be knowledgeable on different types of medication and how they interact as well as the possible side effects of each. As a clinical pharmacist, you get to spend a lot of time interacting with medical professionals and patients and you can also see the patients with a doctor that means that you can participate in analyzing the patient's condition and prescribing medication. A hospital pharmacist on the other hand spends more time in a pharmacy preparing the medication needed by patients.

The main responsibilities of a hospital pharmacist include preparing prescription medication, filling out medical paperwork, providing information needed by medical personnel, making sure that the medication dispensed is safe and fit for patients and ordering as well as monitoring inventory.

### Importance of Clinical Pharmacists

Clinical pharmacists are known to work in direct link with doctors, other professionals in the medical field, and also with patients. They play an important role in ensuring the drugs ordered in prescriptions for patients result in proper outcomes as far as the health of the patients is concerned.

The environment within which clinical pharmacists work is one of health care setting, and as a result they interact regularly not only with doctors but with a range of other health professionals. Through this interaction, the fraternity of health professionals manages to coordinate healthcare services even better.

Clinical pharmacists happen to be well educated and also adequately trained to handle various environments of patient care, where they come into direct contact with the ailing. Among the environments these professionals work are medical centers and clinics, hospitals and other settings where healthcare services are provided. It is normal for pharmacists to be provided with privileges associated with patient care as they collaborate with doctors or different health systems. Such systems permit the pharmacists to do an entire range of functions requiring serious decision making, and they do this as a crucial part of the team of health care providers.

The pharmacists enjoy these privileges out of the fact that they have proven to be knowledgeable in matters of medication therapy, and their record manifests great clinical experience. Such knowledge of a specialized nature as well as impressive clinical experience is gained by way of residence training as well as certification of a specialist board.

### The Role of Clinical Pharmacists

One of the important roles of a clinical pharmacist is to evaluate a patient's health status, and to establish if the medication prescribed meets the needs of that particular patient in an optimal manner. They also seek to establish if the primary goals of care are being met by dispensing the medication prescribed.

Clinical pharmacists also assess how appropriate it is, and also how effective, to provide the said patient with the medications as prescribed. They are prepared to identify any health issues the patient may have but which have not been taken care of; ailments that could be addressed through fitting medication therapy.

Clinical pharmacists may also take up another role of following up on a patient's health progress, so as to establish the effects of medications provided on the given patient's health. It is also their obligation to have consultations with the patient's doctor or other healthcare service providers, so as to identify the medication therapy best for the patient considering all the needs. In short, clinical pharmacists contribute greatly to the overall journey of treatment for the patient.

Another central role of the clinical pharmacist is advising patients on the best way to have their medications. They are also active in supporting the efforts of the entire healthcare providing team in educating patients about important steps they ought to take in order to enhance their health and to maintain it. Examples of areas they participate in giving advice is exercise and diet, and also the area of immunization. These are the areas where, if patients were to heed the advice of clinical pharmacists even as they take their medication, would be greatly improved and the patients' good health, once attained, would be maintained.

Another important role taken up by clinical pharmacists is providing references to patients when it comes to the need for suitable physicians or other therapy providing professionals. This ensures the patients seeing the clinical pharmacists have their health issues properly addressed by experts, and that the medication prescribed is absolutely necessary, in the appropriate dosage and helpful. These pharmacists are even in a position to advice patients on appropriate sources of health available within the social services department.

### How Clinical Pharmacists Ensure Proper Care for Patients

Clinical pharmacists are known to provide care to patients on a consistent basis, and this ensures medication given is timely and appropriate, as well as effective and safe. They also hold consultations with doctors treating the patient as well as other healthcare service providers involved, in a bid to develop a medication plan that is easy to implement for the welfare of the patient. This helps to achieve the goals set for improvement of the patient's care, as well as maintenance of the patient's health with the support and guidance of the healthcare providing team.

Clinical pharmacists are also great sources of expert knowledge, not just for their patients, but also for their colleagues in the healthcare sector. They are resourceful as far as medication related knowledge is concerned, dosing and its appropriateness as well as possible side effects, medication interactions and so on. As such, their contribution as they collaborate with other medical staff to improve health is invaluable.

They also come in handy in urging their colleagues in the medical profession to try solving health issues in a manner that ensures medications are used in a rational manner.

Owing to the relationship clinical pharmacists usually have with their patients, they are often relied upon to provide advice tailored for individual patients. This helps to improve the individual patient's health faster than otherwise, as such a patient's unique needs and inclinations are taken into account.

### Where to Find Clinical Pharmacists

Clinical pharmacists can be found working in different environments, as long as they are areas dealing with improvement of people's health. Often you can find them in hospitals and such other large medical institutions, clinics offering outpatient health services, community based pharmacies, doctor's offices and nursing homes, and even organizations offering managed care.

## Calculation Methods Involving Ratios & Proportions

A ratio can be understood as that relationship existing between some two numbers, which happen to be separated by a colon. A good example is 2:4. This is a ratio whose meaning is that there are two parts of something in every four parts of the other thing in comparison. You can portray the same meaning in a fraction instead of using a ratio. In the example just cited, instead of the ratio, 2:4, you could simply write $\frac{2}{4}$.

As for proportion, is can be defined as an expression involving two ratios that are equal, and the two sets of ratios have what is termed 'means' as well as 'extremities'. Whenever you want to set up some calculation involving ratio and proportion an equals sign separates those two ratios. If the equal sign is not being used, then a double colon, which looks like '::', can be used in its place. A good example is 3:6 = 2:X, which can also be expressed as 3:6 :: 2:X. The term used in reference to the digits on the inside, which in this case are 6 and 2 is 'means', and the term used in reference to the digits on the outer part, in this case 3 and X, is 'extremities'.

Any time you are setting up calculations that involve proportions, you will have at all times known variables and others that are unknown. It is also good to note that among the different variables within calculations involving a ratio and a proportion, at least some variables must be known; in fact, three among the four need to have known values. That is the only way you will be able to solve for the value of the fourth variable. The use of 'X' to represent the unknown variable is typical, otherwise any other letter would work the same.

### Illustration on Ratio/Proportion Working

Solve the following problem of ratio and proportion.

3:6 = 2:X

The value of X = 4

What you do involves multiplication of the means and the multiplication of the extremities, and this way you will easily get the value that is unknown. So, in this case:

6 x 2 = 3 x X.

This means 3x = 12

Hence x = 12 ÷ 3 = 4.

Considering that of the four variables three are already known solving for X should be easy.

Keep in mind the fact you can set up ratios to exist as equations of fractions. For instance, when you have proportions 3:6 = 2:X, as in the previous illustration, you can still turn those ratios into fractions, and once you do that the next step should be to cross multiply. See the example here below.

### Illustration on how to Turn ratio into Fraction

3:6 becomes 3/6

2:X becomes 2/x

Then when you proceed to cross multiply, what you get is:

3/6 x 2/x

3 x X = 3X while 6 x 2 = 12

So you will essentially have 3x = 12, and then you can proceed to solve for x.

Now you need to divide both sides by 3 as your two sides must always remain equal.

3x ÷ 3 = 12 ÷ 3, which works to:

x = 4

### Calculation Methods Involving Dimensional Analysis

This method of Dimensional Analysis or DA, commonly used by pharmacists, is also based on math calculations. You are required to first of all create some pathway of ratio-proportion, and this is on the basis of some combination of quantities provided as well as factors of conversion already known and common in the field of metric calculations and the household measurement system. It is helpful to know the most appropriate time to apply the dimensional analysis method to calculate dosing.

Suppose according the medication record you are required to dispense 1 gram of Azithromycin, and the administration route is oral. It is noted there is need to dispense quantity that is sufficient. However, this particular pharmacy has Azithromycin as tablets of 250mg only. Therefore, the pharmacist has to calculate the number of 250mg tablets of Azithromycin to dispense to the patient.

What is important to know in order to find the correct answer is the number of milligrams there are in a gram, and this is 1,000mg. Besides, you now have the medication in stock and the medication to be dispensed both in like terms. You are now prepared to perform the said dimensional analysis or DA. See illustration below.

## *Illustration of Dimensional Analysis (DA)*

It is known that one gram is comprised of 1,000 milligrams. That is the only conversion necessary for you to succeed in your calculations in such a situation. Or you could have set up the dimensional analysis equation immediately as follows:

1,000mg/1 x 1 tablet/250mg and after you have calculated the product of the numerators divided by the product of the denominators you get 4 tablets.

This is similar to asking how many 250mg tablets would make up 1,000mg, which would require you to simply divide 1,000mg by 250mg to get 4 tablets.

In using DA, it is helpful to form numerators as well as denominators which are easy to cross-cancel each other so that you can be left with the appropriate number of tablets.

## *Dosing Calculations for Liquids and Solids*

Sometimes in the practice of pharmacy, you find some weak solution being made out of a solution that is more concentrated. A good example is some concentrated stock solution. In such instances, the products are usually expressed in terms of percentage weight-volume, or w/v, and in other cases they are expressed in terms of percentage weight-weight, or w/w.

Percent or percentage, as used in the field of pharmacy, denotes the precise number of parts in a hundred parts. For instance, if you have a certain product given as 0.3% w/v, it is supposed to be interpreted to be 0.3 grams (g) in every 100 milliliters (mL). At the same time, if you have a certain product given as 10% w/w, it is supposed to be interpreted to be 10 grams (g) in every 100 grams (g).

There are numerous products available in the market today and they have their concentration stated in either of these formats. A good example is the Fluocinonide solution, which is provided as 0.05% solution. This means that this medication contains 0.05 grams (g) of the drug, fluocinonide, in every 100 milliliters (mL) of the product. There is another good example in 0.1% triamcinolone cream. What the dosage expression means is that the product contains 0.1 grams (g) of the drug, triamcinolone, in each 100 grams (g) of the product.

In some situations, you may realize a given strength is not available when required, or even that the strength of the product available for sale is not suitable, and in actual fact what you need for the patient is a product whose strength is lower than those available. What is done in such situations is that the available product, whose strength is greater than needed, is combined with some diluents that is medically acceptable. If you are calculating dilution of liquids as well as solids, it is important that you apply the appropriate formula.

### *Appropriate Formula in Dilution of Medications*

In case you have solid you want to dilute using some liquid a suitable formula to use is:

Quantity 1 x Concentration 1 = Quantity 2 x Concentration 2

In abbreviated form :

$Q_1$ x $C_1$ = $Q_2$ x $C_2$

Great examples in the use of this math formula are provided here below, and they involve solids and liquids with diluents.

### *Illustration involving Dilution of Liquid Medication*

Calculate the number of milliliters of some 0.4% stock solution when you want to produce 2 liters of some 0.06% solution, and the solvent in use is water.

Workings

You need to recall here that 1 liter is equivalent to 1,000 milliliters.

So as the formula provided can work successfully, you must at any one time have 3 variables with known values. In the situation here, $C_1$ is known to be 0.04%, $Q_2$ is known to be 2 liters, while $C_2$ is known to be 0.06%. As such, the variable whose value is unknown and needs to be calculated is $Q_1$. You will see how to go about solving for it here below.

Keep in mind the need to work with units that are alike when doing calculations. In the situation here, the answer is required in milliliters (mL), and so it is important that the 2 liters be converted to milliliters right away; before embarking on actual calculations.

1,000 milliliters / 1 liter x 2 liters

First of all the liter units cancel out completely, and you will be left with 2 x 1,000 milliliters, and this works out to 2,000 milliliters (mL)

As earlier noted, you have Q1 as unknown; C1 = 0.4%; Q2 = 2000 mL and C2 = 0.06%.

Your workings should therefore be as follows:

0.4 x 100/100 X = 100/100 x 0.06 x 2,000

x = 6/100 x 2,000 x 10/4 = (6 x 20 x 10) ÷ 4

And the answer is 300 milliliters (mL).

In short, you need 300 milliliters of 0.4% stock solution to combine with the liquid. The next step is to find out the number of milliliters of the available solvent you need. In order to establish the exact amount of water, which is the solvent here, is required to add into the compound, you only need to subtract your stock solution volume from what you have as the ultimate volume of the compound.

In this case the volume of compound you ultimately require is 2,000 milliliters, and when you subtract 300 milliliters from it you get:

2,000 mL – 300 mL = 1,700 mL water

Here is a different illustration that involves dilution of a liquid.

Here what you want is to calculate the level of concentration of the solution that has been diluted.

### *Illustration to Calculate Concentration Level*

You have some fresh concentration of 750 milliliters containing a dextrose solution whose level is 50%, and has been diluted with water to make 1,500 milliliters of solution. What this practically means is that:

Q1 = 750; C1 = 50%; Q2 = 1500 mL; C2 = X

Using the same formula as the one in the previous illustration:

Quantity 1 x Concentration 1 = Quantity 2 x Concentration 2

In this case:

750 x 50% = 1,500 x X

1,500X = 375

Therefore X = 0.25 or 25%

Once you dilute the 750 milliliters containing 50% dextrose solution with water so that it becomes 1,500 milliliters, the outcome is a liquid whose concentration of dextrose is now 25%. It is important for you to take note that the amount of active ingredient does not change at all, as you have only doubled the volume of the solution by adding water. In short, while concentration drops, the actual quantity of the important active ingredient remains in the solution to be administered to the patient.

When you want to dilute products that are solid as exemplified by creams or even ointments, the same rules you have followed in the two illustrations above are still the ones you need to follow. Ordinarily you need to use ointments or even bases in diluting products of a solid form, and you should ensure the bases you use have no active drug.

### *Illustration on Dilution of Medication Solids*

Calculate the number of grams of some 5% lidocaine ointment, and also find out the number of grams of ointment base that need to be used to combine with the ointment in order to have 3 pounds of 2% lidocaine treatment.

<u>Workings</u>

It is important to keep in mind that one pound is equivalent to 454 grams. Also note that the formula you used for liquid medications also works well for ointments and other solids. The formula to use, therefore, is:

Quantity 1 x Concentration 1 = Quantity 2 x Concentration 2

Using DA to convert 3 pounds to grams:

3 pounds x 454 grams / 1 pound = 1,362 grams

$Q_1$ x $C_1$ = $Q_2$ x $C_2$

X x 5% = 1,362 x 2%

X = 5% ÷ 1,362 x 2% = 100/5 x 1362 x 2/100

After the two hundreds above and below cancel each other out, you will be left with:

(1,362 x 2) / 5 which works out to 544.8 and you can round it up to 545 grams (g)

In short, you need 545g of 5% lidocaine ointment for the sake of compounding the required product. What you need to do next is find out the amount of base required. Considering it is already known what the ultimate weight of the product will be, which is 1362g, and also that 5% lidocaine ointment of weight 545g is to be used, it is now easy to calculate the base.

Workings

1362 grams – 545 grams = 817 grams of base required.

Here next is a different example that involves dilution of solids. Here you are required to calculate what the ultimate concentration will be as opposed to the actual amounts.

**Illustration to Find Out Concentration**

You have 0.05% Fluocinonide 30 grams ointment to combine with 15 grams of a given ointment base. Calculate the ultimate percentage strength of the diluted solid.

Working

In this illustration, you will be able to see two ways of establishing the required strength.

Using the Concentration Formula

Q1 x C1 = Q2 x C2

Q1 = 30 gm; C1 = 0.05%; Q2 = 45 gm; and C2 = X

30g x 0.05% = 45g x X

X = 30g x 0.05% ÷45g = 30g x 0.05% x 1/45g

100 over a 100 will cancel each other out completely, and when you divide 30g and 45g by 5 you remain with 6 and 9 respectively. So you now have:

(6 x 0.05%)/9 which works out to 0.3%/9= 0.333% or simply 0.03% concentration.

As such, the renewed percentage strength of the medication, fluocinonide, is 0.03%.

There is also a different way of finding out the renewed percentage strength of fluocinonide, and this is the ratio-proportion way. You can see the illustration here below.

Workings

Remember originally the concentration of the medication was 0.05% and this means there was 0.05 grams of the drug, fluocinonide, in the 100 grams of the substance. On the basis of this clear information, find out the number of fluocinonide grams there are within 30 grams of the substance.

<u>Workings</u>

This is how the proportion method works

0.05 grams/100 grams = x/30grams which is 0.05 x 30 = 100x

Therefore, x = 0.015 grams (g)

Now you know X = 0.015 grams, and this is to say 0.015 grams of the drug, fluocinonide, are within the tube of 30 grams. The next step will be to find out the strength of the product now in percentage, and this is after the addition of 15 grams of the ointment base. Remember the quantity of active ingredient does not change, and instead what changes is the overall weight of the product, because it is now 45 grams.

0.015 grams/45 grams = x/100 grams

This works out to:

45 grams x X = 0.015 x 100, which leads to X = (0.015 x 100)/45 which becomes 0.0333 or 0.03%

### *Aliquot as a Measure*

In the practice of pharmacy, you find cases where the quantity of drug required is very tiny, and this becomes a problem in so far as measuring the drug is concerned. The devices normally in use, even for small amounts, like balances or even graduated cylinders are not fit enough for such tiny amounts, as they happen to have what is termed MWQ or minimum weighable quantity, and sometimes MMQ or minimum measurable quantity.If this MWQ or MMQ is already higher than the quantity required, then certainly measuring such a quantity becomes a challenge.

### *Illustration on Using the Aliquot*

You have a compound that needs 20 milligrams of codeine, yet the drug available has MWQ of 120 milligrams. As such, it is impossible to measure the 20 milligrams required out of the 120 milligrams of the drug. What is used in such instances is an aliquot.

By aliquot is actually meant having exactly some given number of times in relation to something different, and it is the best way to measure amounts that are very tiny. It also means that in case you divide that factor within the quantity, nothing remains; so in your calculation you do not get a remainder. In the field of pharmacy, you use this method of aliquot to measure some tiny amount of a given chemical or even drug, and this you do by diluting some amount that is larger than the needed, and that ends up making it possible to acquire the amount required even if it is tiny. You can see this in the example here below.

### *Illustration on Using the Aliquot*

Set aside 100 milliliters of 0.3 milligrams per milliliter clonidine (mg/mL) solution, and use water as your diluents.

Workings

The first step should be to find out the amount of clonidine required.

0.3 milligrams/1 milliliters x 100 milliliters = 30 milligrams clonidine

If you make the assumption that MWQ for the medication remaining and available is 120 milligrams, then, obviously, 30 milligrams is not possible to measure. In this case, therefore, you can only use the aliquot.

It is crucial that the quantities to be measured be identified with keenness, so that they are neither too large as to waste resources. In this case, it is evident 120 milligrams is the amount that can be measured at the minimum, and so it is the quantity of clonidine that will be used here. Keep in mind the aliquot will also require measuring, and you can take 5 milliliters to be the aliquot volume.

As such, considering ultimately what needs to be measured is 30 milligrams of clonidine, the aliquot concentration will be taken to be 30 milligrams per 5 milliliters. You can proceed to perform this as a proportion, in determining the required volume meant to dilute 120 milligrams clonidine in form of 30 milligrams per milliliter of concentration.

30 milligrams/5 milliliters = 120 milligrams/x

After cross multiplying, you get:

30x = 120 x 5 or 30x = 600

Therefore, x = 600 ÷ 30 = 20

In order to acquire 30 milligrams of clonidine that is required to make the compound, you need to first ensure dilution of 120 milligrams of the drug, clonidine using 20 milliliters of water. Next, you need to proceed to measure 5 milliliters aliquot and then embark on diluting until you reach the ultimate volume which is 100 milliliters. This method of calculation works pretty well with substances whose dosage is in solid form, and requiring inert diluents like lactose.

### *Alligation as a Measurement Method*

Alligation can be described as some method involving the mixing of solutions or solids that are similar, in the process of calculating a given percentage strength that you cannot acquire through normal supplies. You can also use this method when the drug amount you need is not readily available at the pharmacy.

# Chapter 10: Proper Medication Administration

Medication plays a major role in diagnosing, treating as well as preventing diseases. You can take medication in all manner of forms including injection, tablets, solution and in many other forms and the mode in which you administer the medication also varies depending on the form of the medicine. You can either administer the medication yourself or have a health care provider do it for you. Some medication such as injections for diabetic persons can also be done by a family member or trained persons at home.

Ideally, drugs are meant to treat or improve your health but they can also become dangerous and sometimes even life threatening when they are administered in the wrong way. It is therefore important for you to learn how to use medication correctly as prescribed by your medical care provider.

### *Various Routes of Administering Medication*

There are three major factors that determine how a drug should be administered in the body. These three factors include the formula or form of the medication, the way in which the drug does its work in the body and the part in the body which is being treated. For example, some drugs are likely to destroy the digestive system in the body when taken orally and so they have to be given through injection while others should be applied topically to the skin because of the area in the body that they are required to treat.

There are a number of routes through which you can administer medication into the body depending on the factors we have listed above. For example, there are drugs which are administered into the body through a slightly invasive way such as enteral medication which is delivered into your intestines or stomach directly using a J-tube or a G-tube and rectal medication which is inserted into your rectum.

Others are less invasive than the enteral and rectal medication such as infused medication which is slowly injected over time into your veins using IV lines, intramuscular medication which is injected into your muscles using syringes, intrathecal which enters your spine through injection and intravenous medication that is injected into IV lines or directly into your veins.

Some drugs are given through the nose such as inhalable medication which is breathed in with the help of a mask or tube and nasal drugs which are administered into the nose through spraying or pumping. Other drugs are administered through the mouth such as buccal drugs which are held inside your cheek, sublingual drugs which are held under your tongue and oral medications which are swallowed through the mouth in form of capsules, tablets, liquid or lozenges.

There are drugs that are administered into your body through the skin such as subcutaneous medication which is injected just below the skin, topical drugs that are applied directly onto your skin and transdermal drugs which are given through placing a patch onto the skin. Other drugs such as otic drugs are given by putting drops in the ear while others such as ophthalmic drugs are administered into the eye through ointment, gels and eye drops.

### Techniques of Medication Administration

In most cases, you can administer medication to yourself at your home or have a family member or anyone who can follow directions do it for you. However, there are certain medications that should be administered by professionally trained health care givers such as nurses, doctors and other trained professionals due to the risks involved if the medication is not given in the correct way.

Administering medication requires you to have a thorough understanding of the drug. Some of the important things that you should know include how a drug works and moves in the body, the correct way it should be administered, the potential side effects as well as any dangerous reactions that can occur and how to store, handle and dispose it.

Health care givers go through rigorous training on all the above issues to ensure that there are as few medication errors as possible. There are "five rights" that you should consider when handling medication. These are the correct patient, the correct drug, the correct time, the correct dose and the correct route.

However, despite having trained health care providers, medical errors are often reported. It is recorded that medication errors account for about 1.4 million injuries reported each year in the United States. This can be greatly attributed to health care providers not following the "five rights" of handling medication to the letter. These "rights" when followed can be the starting point of ensuring that medication is handled correctly and injuries reported due to medical errors are significantly reduced.

### Importance of Dosage and Dispensing Timing

It is important for you to give medication doses exactly as it is advised on the prescription and follow all the directions as indicated. Doctors carefully determine what dosage to prescribe for each patient depending on factors such as a patient's weight, age, liver and kidney health as well as other health factors.

For some medication however, a doctor can only determine the correct dosage through trial and error. So that they can finally determine the correct dosage that a patient needs in this manner, they need to closely monitor you especially on the first trial when they start administering the medication. For example, when the doctor prescribes blood thinners or thyroid medication, you may find that you will be required to take regular blood and urine tests over the period that you are on medication to determine whether the dose is too low or too high. These test results can help the doctor determine how much adjustment they need to make to your dosage up to that point where they finally have the right dosage for you.

Medication is required to get to certain levels in the bloodstream for it to start working as expected. This is why drugs should be administered at specified times in the day and after a specific number of hours so that the required level of medication in the bloodstream can be maintained. The level of medication in the system can be too low to work as it is required when you take medication later than you should and too high than is required when you take it sooner than you should and so you need to maintain the correct balance for it to work effectively.

### *Need to Express Potential for Drug Problems*

It is also important for you to inform your doctor of any medication that you are taking to avoid a reaction between the drugs you are taking and those that you are about to be put on. If you have had any kind of allergic reaction to any drug or foods in the past or if you have an existing allergic reaction to anything, it is also important to notify your doctor. Many unwanted effects of medication happen because of lack of open communication between the doctor and the patient and so it is necessary for you to give any information that is necessary to your doctor.

Some drugs can have adverse effects on you and so they can only be administered by a doctor. In some few cases, you may be required to stay in the health facility during this period so that your doctor can monitor you and see how the medication reacts with your body. When taking medication yourself, it is your responsibility to look out for any side effects such as swelling, rashes, dizziness, fatigue, vomiting and other possible problems and you need to notify your doctor immediately if you experience any serious effects.

You should make sure that you take all medication correctly as prescribed by your doctor and using the "five rights" ensure that it is the right drug, taken at the right time, in the right dose and using the right route. If someone else is administering the drug on your behalf then ensure that they follow the same rules.

If there are any questions you need to ask your doctor regarding your medication, do so and ensure that you completely understand all the necessary details about your drugs. Some of the important questions you need to ask your doctor may include how often you should take your medication, what kind of side effects you should look out for, the time in the day you are required to take your drugs and whether it is necessary that you take them at that particular time. If you are not able to take your medication by yourself, you can also ask your doctor if it is okay for a health care giver or someone in your family to give it to you. If a healthcare giver is the one who administers your medication but you would want to do it for yourself then you can also ask if it is okay to do so and whether you can be trained on how to give it. If you are on any other medication, you can also ask your doctor whether this will cause a negative reaction when combined with other drugs.

It is vital to take the correct dosage as prescribed by your doctor so that it can be effective in treating or managing illness but failure to do so can cause a lot of harm and sometimes even threaten life. For example, when your doctor prescribes antibiotics, you need to ensure that you take the right dose and at the right time so that the level of medication needed in your bloodstream can remain constant. If you fail to do this, your infection might become worse or become entirely unresponsive to the medication and even after the infection is gone, you should complete the dose to avoid recurring.

Some drugs can cause a lot of harm if you consume more than is required and opiod pain drugs such as codeine and oxycodone fall into that category. Taking too much of these drugs can cause addiction and in some cases they can even cause death. In general, all drugs are designed to treat, prevent and manage diseases but they can be potentially dangerous if you abuse them.

### Subcutaneous Injection

This is a form of giving medication that involves injecting the drug under your skin. For you to get the medicine into your body, you are required to inject it in between the inner layer of your skin and your muscles using a needle. Medication that is given in this manner takes a longer time to be absorbed into the body unlike when you inject it directly into your veins.

This method of injecting is often used when any other methods are considered less effective or harmful. For instance, the enzymes and acids found in your stomach can destroy some drugs before they even have a chance to work. Other ways of administering such as intravenous injections may be too costly or difficult and so subcutaneous injections becomes the ideal method of administering the drug into the body.

Medications that are given in very small amounts of about 1ml to 3 ml such as insulin and several types of hormones are mostly given through subcutaneous injection. Drugs that require to be administered very quickly are also candidates for this method of administration such as epinephrine which is used to treat serious allergic reactions.

Epinephrine is packaged in a tube with an automatic injector known as an EpiPen that is quickly stabbed into a patient's thigh or arm during an attack.

Other drugs that can be given through subcutaneous injection include pain medication such as hydromorphone (Dillaudid) and morphine as well as drugs used to prevent vomiting and nausea such as dexamethasone (DexPak) and metoclopramide (Reglan.) Some allergy shots and vaccines can be administered through subcutaneous injection although most of them are given through intramuscular injection.

When you are getting subcutaneous injections, it is crucial for the doctor to know what part of the body to inject. Usually, the injection should be done into the fatty tissue which is just below your skin. There are certain areas of your body where the layers of tissue are more accessible and this is the ideal place to have the injection because the chances of hitting a muscle, blood vessel or bone are thin. The three most common places you can receive injection are the front part of your thigh, the side or back of your upper arm and the abdomen right under the belly button.

For you to receive an injection, the doctor needs to have three main things. These are the medication stored in vials, syringes with short needles of about five eighth inches long and an auto-injector pen. The needle should have a thickness of about 27 or 28 gauge with a length of not more than six eighth. However patients who require a dose of more than 3ml or people who have eyesight problems may need a different kind of needle.

### *Buccal and Sublingual Medication Administration*

Buccal and sublingual methods of administration involve giving medication through the mouth. Buccal administration refers to the process of administering medication by placing the medicine between your cheek and gum while sublingual administration refers to the process of administering medication by placing the medicine under the tongue. In both cases, the drug dissolves and it is slowly absorbed into the blood stream through the mouth tissue. The area under your tongue as well as your cheek area has small blood vessels and many capillaries that absorb the drugs directly into the bloodstream. Medication given in such methods is usually in film, spray or tablet form.

Your doctor can prescribe the buccal or sublingual methods of administration in circumstances such as when the medicine needs to be absorbed into your body quickly, when the medicine is not absorbed well in your stomach, when you have difficulties in swallowing medication or when the digestive process in your stomach will lessen the effectiveness of the medication when swallowed.

### Benefits of Buccal and Sublingual Drug Administration

There are several advantages associated with taking drugs using the buccal and sublingual methods. One of them is that in case of an emergency such as a heart attack, a doctor can give medicine through these methods because it is absorbed into your blood stream quickly. If you have difficulties in swallowing pills then these methods are ideal for you because all you have to do is place the drug in your mouth and wait for it to dissolve. Another advantage is that you can take a slightly lower dose of medication and get similar results as someone who takes it orally because these methods do not involve your digestive system meaning that they are not metabolized through the liver.

### Disadvantages of Buccal and Sublingual Drug Administration

When you eat, drink or smoke when administering the drug, there is a high chance that it will not work as effectively as it should because this will alter the way the medication is absorbed into the bloodstream. Another disadvantage is that any cuts or open sores inside your mouth may be irritated by medication leading to great discomfort or even pain. Some medications like extended-release formulations are supposed to be processed slowly in the system and so such methods are not ideal for this kind of medication.

It is advisable to tell your care giver if you are a smoker or have any open sores or cuts in the mouth before they prescribe buccal or sublingual medication. You should also ask the doctor for what period of time you are required to stay without eating or drinking after you have taken medication. In some cases, you are required to go for hours without consuming anything and so it is important to be informed.

### The Transdermal Patch

This is a patch which contains medication which works by attaching the patch onto your skin. The drug found in this patch is then absorbed into the body over time. This is a good alternative for you if you are not comfortable with taking pills or receiving an injection. Some of the common drugs administered in patches are clonidine which is used to manage high blood pressure, fentanyl which is a pain reliever and nicotine which helps smokers to quit smoking.

### About Intravenous Medication Administration

Intravenous is a medical term that simply means 'into the vein'. Intravenous medication administration is a process used to deliver an injection or liquid substances into the body through the veins. By the use of a tube or a needle, these substances are delivered to the body through a process commonly known as drips.

IV administration is the fastest way to deliver medications by using atube called the catheter that is injected into your vein. This catheter can be used for delivering medications, fluid replacement, blood transfusions etc.

The healthcare providers do not allow anybody to administer self IV treatment. This is because safety and hygiene of the catheter must be highly maintained to avoid infection.

Although some patients have been allowed to use them at home, most are likely to receive this type of medical administration from a hospital. The IV medication administration provides a safe administration of medication without having needles poking at you every time especially if you are getting a prolonged treatment.

### Uses of IV medications

Using the IV administration is critical in most medical cases due to its efficiency and accuracy. There are various cases whereby the IV medication becomes the only best method to administer the required treatment. Such cases include:

During emergency cases, the IV medication is administered to manage the situation in the fastest way possible. Administering pills or liquid medicine by mouth during such instances is not quick enough to save a life.

IV administration ensures the medication goes straight into the blood stream quickly sending the required help to the necessary organs. Through the use of the IV catheter, the doctors are able to adjust and provide the right dosage of the medication.

There are certain medicines that can only be administered through the IV process due to the nature of their absorption. If such medicines are taken orally, they are hindered by the enzymes in the stomach from working as they should. Therefore, the IV administration becomes more effective in administering such drugs.

In cases where a patient needs to be under constant medication, the IV provides the best administration in a friendly controlled manner.

### About standard IV lines

Intravenous lines are different and are categorized according to which vein the inserted catheter empties into.

Standard lines are the most common IV lines that are useful for short hospital stays. For example, in eliminating pain, nausea or administering antibiotics for a short period of time, a standard IV is line is used.

Standard IV lines are used for about four days. Any hospital stay that prolongs the four days sees the IV line changed into something else that will cater for the longer stay.

When administering a standard IV line, a needle is injectedtoa vein found on the backside of a hand or your elbow or your wrist. The IV tube is inserted over a needle, as a needle is pulled out leaving the catheter sitting in place. To ensure itsits perfectly, you can get use a small band to fasten the catheter. This also stops the bleeding that occurs when the catheter is pushed into your vein.

A standard IV line is commonly used for 2typesof administration. These include:

### IV Infusion

This is administration that happens over time and requires controlled medication release into the bloodstream. The IV infusion either uses pump or gravity to send medication into the catheter. It has two methods of administration that include:

### Drip infusion

This is the most common kind of IV infusion you can find almost anywhere. It uses gravity to deliver the required amount of medication continually over a required period of time. A drip, commonly placed next to a patient allows the medication to slowly flow through the tube into the catheter right into the blood stream.

### Pump infusion

Also commonly found especially in the US, the pump infusion is joined to the Intravenous line which dispenses the medication slowly but steadily. Pump infusion is mostly used to make sure the dosage needs to be very accurate and controlled.

### IV Push

This mode of administration is a quick injection of medication into the catheter to send a one-time dose into your bloodstream. It is commonly used to curb intense pain or administer antibiotic to stop a certain reaction in the body fast enough.

### Types Of Central Venous Catheters

With standard IV lines administering short term medication, there are other lines that deliver long term treatment like chemotherapy and the like. Such long term IV administration needs a central venous catheter (CVC).

The CVC is commonly inserted to a major vein on your neck, arm, groin area or chest. A CVC stays in place for a long time and can last for weeks or months of your stay in hospital.

There are three key types of Central Venous Catheters that are commonly used. They include:

### Tunneled catheter

A tunneled catheter allows medication to be directed into the blood vessels of the heart. It is commonly used during surgical procedures whereby the IV is placed in the chest or neck of the patient. The other part of the IV line is channeled through the entire body and its end comes out via the skin. This end of the catheter is where the medication is administered into the blood stream.

### (PICC) Peripherally inserted central catheter

The Peripherally Inserted Central Catheter is placed in a vein that is above your elbow on your upper side of the arm. It is a long line that sends the required medication from the insertion area through the blood vessels to a vein near your heart.

### Implanted Port

A port that is implanted works the same as a tunneled catheter although their insertion is a bit different. It is used during short surgical procedures. It is inserted into a vein in the chest or neck and slid under the skin. The medication is then injected under the skin to the port on the IV line implanted beneath the skin. This directs the drugs into the blood as required.

### Drugs Typically Given By IV

Different kinds of treatments are administered differently. IV being one of the best methods to administer medications has special prescriptions it delivers. Some of these medications include:

Pain relief medications like the morphine and hydromorphone

- Antibiotics medications like the gentamicin, vancomycin and meropenem

- Chemotherapy medications like the cisplatin, vincristine, paclitaxel and doxorubicin

- Antifungal medications like amphotericin and micafungin

- Immunoglobulin medications

- Low blood pressure medications like dobutamine, dopamine, norepinephrine, and epinephrine.

### Possible IV Side effects

Although IV medication has been termed as generally safe for use for the longest time, it has been proved to cause some side effects that are either mild or dangerous. Every medication administered through the IV line reaches the body fast using the blood stream.

On reaching the body, they also act very fast to suppress whatever condition the body is fighting. Side effects are therefore experienced from hypersensitive reactions and additional effects that happen as fast also. In severe cases, a patient develops an allergic reaction during the infusion or immediately after. That's why the healthcare provider always observesthe patient keenly to note any side effects.

### Examples of IV side effects may include:

### Injury to vessels of the blood or Site of injection

During the injection or while inserting the catheter line, a vein could be injured. This damage causes infiltration meaning the medication trickles into the surrounding area instead of entering into the blood vessels as required. Infiltration is known to cause tissue impairment.

Other damages caused to the blood vessels are veins inflammation and phlebitis. Phlebitis and infiltration have similar symptoms that include pain, puffiness at the jabarea and warmth that is a discomfort. If you notice any one of these indications it is wise to inform the doctor.

### Chances of Air embolism

During the insertion of the needle and the catheter line, it is important to ensure no enters the needle or to the IV treatment bag. This is because the air can make the line run dry allowing the air bubbles to enter into your vein.

The danger comes when the air bubbles move to your lungs or heart and cause a blood flow blockage. This can cause seriouscomplications such as a stroke or a heart attack.

This is one of the greatest reason why IV administration is only carried out in hospitals by professionals.

### Potential for Blood clots

During the insertion of the IV line, blood flows out from the pricked vein. If a blood clot forms in the vein, it blocks significant blood veins and causes major tissue damage that could lead to death. Another dangerous problem that comes out of a blood clot is the Deep vein thrombosis that can be caused by IV treatments.

### Possibility of Infection

Most infection of the IV administration occur at the injection area. To prevent such kinds of infections from occurring, the healthcare giver always ensures that the process is done in a highly hygienic condition using sterile equipment.

The danger of this infection is the fact that it can travel through the blood stream causing a severe infection throughout the body. Symptoms to check out for in case of an infection include: chills and fevers, pain, swelling and redness of the injection area. If you noticeany of these symptoms, contact your doctor right away before it's too late.

### About Intravenous Fluid Regulation

IV medication administration is carried out for numerous reasons. All these reasons control the amount and type administered. Intravenous Fluid regulation is a regulator of the exact amount of medication that you should receive.

Without the Intravenous fluid regulation, the amount of the fluid or medication being administered can end up receiving too little or too much because it relies on gravity alone to flow.

That's why the regulation is highly maintained either using manual methods or by use of some electric pump. Health care givers must always check the IV to ensure it is properly regulated to provide the flow and conveyance of the accurate usage. This ensures the patient are not put in any danger while receiving the IV administration.

### Importance Of IV Fluid Regulation

As stated above, it is important to ensure the right amount of fluid is being received through the IV line. There are some treatments that heavily count on an IV delivery from the beginning to the end. These include:

Management of pain using some kind of medications

Cancer management through the chemotherapy medications

Rehydration after an illness that caused too much dehydration

### Infection Treatment Using Antibiotics

Fluids for these kind of treatments consist water with sugar, medications, electrolytes that are added in concentrate forms depending on the need of the patient. The rate at which the intravenous quantity is administered depends on the age, medical condition as well as body weight and size.

Regulation ensures that the precisequantity of fluid is dispensed into the IV vein in the accurate rate. Remember complications results both from deliveryof too little too slowly or too much too quickly. This should be highly monitored to eliminate any kind of danger.

### Various Kinds Of Intravenous Fluid Regulation

Having learned the need to controlthe quantity of the fluids flowing at any given time, it is important to learn the two ways this can be done – manually or by use of an electric pump. These two methods require a healthcare provider to check and ascertain that you are receiving the rightquantity of medication. Let's look at the two ways to regulate the IV.

### Electric pump regulation

This regulation is much easier than the manual one. The nurse simply programs the pump to administer the desired amount of fluid into the IV tube at a controlled rate.

### Manual regulation

This is simply done by manually increasing or decreasing the pressure of the fluid flow. A clamp is the point that puts the IV tube on check by allowing either a slow or high speed level of flow. The healthcare provider counts the amount of dropletseach minute to ensure the flow rate is accurate and adjusts where needed.

### What To Expect As Procedure Is Undertaken

The IV administration is a procedure that only healthcare professionals should handle.A doctor should always first define the kind of fluid the patient needs for treatment, the duration and the amount needed. The level at which it is delivered is also included to the duration to give a clear statement of both.

A nurse then disinfects the patient's skin area where the injection will go through to ensure it is hygienically clean. The nurse traces the vein that will be used and inserts the IV tube into it. It has a little sting during insertion but should not hurt after that.

Once the catheter tube is inserted, the nurse regulates the flow either by use of pump or manually to program it according to the right flow rate. The same nurse or a different one will need to check the patient regularly to ensure it's all working well. If any problems are noted on the flow, it is adjusted for best results.

### *Possible complications of IV fluid regulation*

Intravenous fluid regulation helps the doctor deliver the right amount of medication and the patient receive the right kind of treatment. However, in the history of the regulation, there are a few minor risks associated with the directive of treatments.

These include:

- A lot of fluid; too quickly causing a fluid overload

- Too little fluid that is released too gradually

Fluid overload can be easily detected through its symptoms that include: headache, anxiety, trouble breathing and high blood pressure. Some of these symptoms could be mild allowing you to tolerate the reaction if you are strong and healthy. It could be dangerous if you suffer from other underlying health problems. To ensure you are safe, report any symptom experienced during the IV administration to your doctor immediately.

Too little fluid causes a low flow speed that causes the patient to delay in responding to the treatment administered. The signs of a slow flow level may vary from person to person but the most outstanding symptom is lack of response or slow response to treatment as expected by the doctor.

The IV administration is safe and efficient. However, if you sight the flow is either too slow or too fast, simply ask your healthcare provider to confirm the flow level. If you also experience any symptoms that you do not understand what is causing it, better still alert your doctor or nurse.

### *Use of the Infusion Pump*

An infusion pump is a health tool used to administer fluids to the patient's body in a more regulated manner. These pumps are commonly found in the hospitals, clinical homes and hospitals.

Infusion pumps are able to deliver both large and small amounts of fluids. Therefore they are used to administer medications as well as nutrients. An infusion pump must be activated by a skilled user who plans the flow speed and a period of the fluid delivery.

Generally infusion pumps give better services than their manual counterparts through their ability to be programmed or automated as the need requires. They are able to deliver medications like hormones, antibiotics, pain relievers as well as chemotherapy drugs.

There are various different kinds of mixture pumps that include large volume pumps, insulin pumps, and patientdirected analgesia, syringe, elastomeric and enteral pumps.Some of these infusion pumps are designed to be stationary used at the bedside of the patient while others are known as ambulatory pumps are wearable or portable.

Pump failures could be detrimental to a patient who is relying on it for their health. That's why they are designed with special features that help patients remain safe by reporting the failure through the fitted features.

Due to the nature of work these pumps do, to give critical fluids and high threat medications, they are fitted with security features like operator alerts and alarms that are meant to trigger in case of a difficulty.

For instance, some older pumps have features that alert consumers when air or anything else blocks the tube. The newer version also known as smart pumps is even better fitted with features that detect an opposing drug reaction, or settings that are set outside of the specified limits.

All these features help both the doctor and the patient regulate the right fluids administered at all times.

**Common IV Types**

A human body is 60% water! Most of the water, about 2/3 is kept intracellular. Most if not all patients who visit the hospital seeking any kind of treatment has to have their hydration status addressed as the first thing.

There are numerous kinds of IV solutions the doctors may select from on condition of the patient's account and diagnosis. In most cases the commonly used fluids are colloids and crystalloids.

Colloids are fluids that have huge particles which linger in the extracellular surface therefore drawing water from the cells and keeping it in the plasma.

Crystalloids are fluids that contain small elements that could pass easily through the cellular membrane. The crystalloids are isotonic, hypotonic, or hypertonic. This write up focuses more on the crystalloids because they are the commonly used IV fluids out of the two.

Four most common IV solutions you may see in the IV department are:

### *About Lactated Ringers*

These are also referred to as LR, RL or even Ringers Lactate. Lactated Ringers is an isotonic crystalloid solution that comprises of potassium chloride, sodium chloride, sodium lactate and calcium chloride in sterile water. It is mostly comparable to the body's serum and plasma concentration.

This solution is outstanding for burn patients or those who have hypovolemia problems due to the fluid shifts. Patients with liver problems should avoid this solution by all means because the liver will not be able to process the lactate bringing more problems to the body.

### *9% Normal Saline*

Sometimes it is also referred to as NS, NSS or even 0.9NaCl. This mixture is better known as isotonic saline or physiological saline. It is less common compared to other IV solutions. This fluid is used for hydration needs for vomiting, hemorrhage, diarrhea or shock. It is one of the best fluid for resuscitation needs.

Normal saline comprises 0.9% sodium chloride that is dissolved in sterilized water. It is a fluid that is used alongside most blood administration processes. With patients who are suffering from any cardiac or renal concession, it should be used with caution or completely avoided due to the high levels of sodium that could cause fluid holding that could put more pressure on the kidneys and the heart.

### *5% Dextrose in Water*

This is also sometimes presented as D5 or even D5W). D5 is an isotonic sugar mixture that comprises of glucose being the solute. This solution when absorbed allows the glucose to quickly grab up the cells and utilize them for vigor, leaving water only which is a hypotonic mixture.

D5W offers 170 calories for every liter which is much needed energy by diabetic patients. This solution is avoided by patients who have renal failure, intracranial pressure and cardiac patients since it can cause fluid overload. Renal and cerebral edema patients cannot undertake the fluid overload of tissues therefore should avoid this solution by all means.

### 45% Normal Saline

Sometimes it is also referred to as Half Normal Saline, 0.45NaCl). Normal saline is a hypotonic crystalloid fluid that is made up of sodium chloride in disinfected water. It is not a normal 0.9% saline solution rather it is a fluid with a higher level of sodium concentration.

This solution is used to give cellular dehydration that is triggered by conditions as diabetic ketoacidosis and hypernatremia. Burn patients, liver patients and trauma patients must avoid this solution by all means because it has aninclination to reduce the intravascular fluid making it dangerous for such patients.

Half standard saline water causes a shift of water from that extracellular liquid area to the ICF section.

### About the Intravenous Intermittent Infusion

Triple III or Intravenous Intermittent Infusion is a mixture that has a volume of liquid as well as medication that are administered during a span of time at timed breaks and stopped till the next dosage is essential.

An irregular infusion may also be known as piggyback treatment, a mini bag mediation or a secondary medication. This infusion maybe given in lesser amounts of disinfected IV fluids whose dosage is 25- 250 ml, which is mixed over an anticipated time just as single dose.

Most medications need to be administered gradually to avoid any abrupt reaction on the patient. This slow technique of administration decreases the high danger of quick mixture. A given piggyback treatment is administered through a recognized IV line which is patented by some solution that is incessant.

Be sure to check every time the parental Therapy Manual to guarantee that the precise directions are adhered to each time a specific medication is given. This particular manual gives you the proper guidelines to combine the IV solutions, the quantity and kind of solutions as well as the ratio of mixing.

Intermittent Medication can also be delivered by either electronic infusion device (EID) commonly known as infusion pump or by gravity. The piggyback IV treatments must always be go together with an Intravenous pump that call for programming and dedicated training to avoid any treatment faults.

The IV infusion pumps offer both soft and hard dosage limits as well as safety training guidelines that help in ensuring safe treatment administration is practiced. IV treatments may be also prepared through gravity mixture. In this case the doctor must analyze the infusion speed – droplets per minute to ensure it is accurately administered. The best preparation for the piggyback mixtures is to have an IV Infusion pump.

### Guidelines For The Intravenous Fluid Therapy

Inpatient or hospitalized patients require IV solution as well as electrolytes for the following reasons:

### Routine maintenance

Routine maintenance means that some patients may require the IV solutions because it is not possible for them to fulfill their electrolyte or normal fluid needs orally or by enteral routes. This may mean they are even weak in comparison to the electrolyte and balance of the fluid, but have no noteworthy deficits, redistribution issues and ongoing irregular losses.

When such a case of routine maintenance is presented, it is important to fulfill the patient's requests for such maintenance while regulating the upkeep prescription to be more accountable for the complex treatment or electrolyte issues. Requirements for the routine maintenance are highly important for every patient who are on ongoing IV solution therapy.

### Fluid resuscitation

IV solutions are given instantly to reinstate circulation to important organs following loss of intravascular capacity due to plasma loss, bleeding or extreme external fluid and electrolyte loss. This is usually from severe internal losses or gastrointestinal tract or severe internal losses.

### Redistribution

Most patients in the hospital are marked with an abnormal fluid handling or internal fluid distribution problems. This problem is mostly seen in patients who are seriously ill, post-surgery patients, major liver, cardiac or renal patients.

Many of the patients get edema from excess water and sodium fluids in the perinatal cavities or the GI tract. Choosing the right amount, rate of management and composition of the IV solutions that will address these complex cases is a difficult assessment. Yet in common admission, both prescribing as well as monitoring the IV solutions is majorly left to the low-ranking doctors and nurses who lack the compulsory training and skill.

There is enough evidence suggesting mismanagement of solutions is quite common especially in the common wards with high risk of long stays at the hospice, additional morbidity as well as mortality as well as increased costs.

That said, there is need for direction on how the IV treatment is prescribed and applied to all general ward patients. Since the greatest randomized well-ordered trials involving IV solution therapy have only been undertaken in the intensive care, many endorsements for the total usage must be founded on the first values.

All health experts who are involved in the administering and prescribing IV fluids ought to fully understand the principles to follow in managing the IV fluid treatment and prescription effectively and safely.

### Replacement

In cases where the patients do not require intravascular or other fluid compartment, they are still required to correct electrolyte or existing water deficits or any continual external losses.

These losses come from common cases like the Urinary tract or the GI. These losses may appear with no much signs while others usually occur with fever like burns that can result to loss of high quantity of plasma.

Most times these deficits develop very slowly and have associated compensatory adaptations of fluid distribution as well as tissue electrolyte that must always be taken into account in the succeeding replacement regimens.

### Set Procedures for prescribing Fluids

The wisdom needed to decode how to effectively administer IV electrolyte and fluid is described in four parts:

- The features of available IV fluids

- The physiology of solution stability in health

- Clinical methods to evaluating IV fluid needs

- Pathophysiological properties on fluid stability.

### The Intramuscular Injection

This is an injection technique that is used to administer medication into your muscles allowing it to become absorbed quickly into your bloodstream. Some of the common medications given through intramuscular injections include vaccines such as a flu shot. You can self- administer intramuscular injections for conditions such as rheumatoid arthritis and multiple sclerosis.

Intramuscular injections can be used when all other methods of administration such as oral administration, intravenous injections and subcutaneous injections are not recommended. Sometimes it can be hard to locate a vein when using intravenous injections and sometimes also, the injection can cause irritation to the veins and so in such circumstances you can opt for an intramuscular injection. Some drugs can also be altered by the acid and enzymes found in your digestive system and so intramuscular injections become a safer option over taking oral medication.

### Targeting the Arm's Deltoid Muscle

The most common area you can receive an intramuscular injection is the deltoid muscle. However, it is not easy for you to self inject on this area and so you may require help from a care giver or a family member. For you to locate the deltoid muscle, you should feel for the bone that is situated at the upper part of your upper arm. For you to inject the correct spot, you should place three fingers right below your acromion process and there below your fingers there will be triangular shape and that is where you should have the injection.

### Vastus Lateralis Muscle of the thigh

You can use the thigh especially when you are administering the injection by yourself because it is a visible site and your risk of causing an error is lower.

### Ventrogluteal Muscle of the hip

This is so far the safest place to inject for both children and adults because it is not near any major nerves or blood vessels. The only disadvantage you have with this site is that it is difficult to self inject and so you may require help from a friend, care giver or family member.

### Dorsogluteal Muscle of the buttocks

For many years, this was the preferred injection site by care givers but over time the Ventrogluteal Muscle has become the more common site for intramuscular injections because of the risk involved with injuring the sciatic muscle. It is also not an ideal location for self-injecting.

### The Drip Bar of Modern Day

Most people who end up on hospital beds or emergency rooms have one fear in common – receiving an IV tube in their veins. Fear of needles rules across the world with no one in particular looking forward to the intravenous catheter installed in their body.

IV tubes are painless but the original needle stick is painful especially once the needle fails to get into the right vein and it requires numerous attempts to get it. IV's have never been personally demanded for but they have been prescribed in so many cases to grant survival.

From cases of failing digestive system, to receiving blood transfusions, to getting more solutions than you can drink, to getting medication that cannot be orally consumed to a range of other prescriptions, IV's have been medically required for many different tasks. In critical cases where there could be massive bleeding, dangerous low blood pressure, devastating infections, IV fluids have dramatically almost miraculously saved lives and increased the chances of surviving.

### Interesting Trend Developing – IVs on demand

In many places especially in the US you can personally ask for an IV fluid and you will get it. This is a new trend that has not been there in the past – the doctors have always done the prescription part and the patient received what the doctor prescribed. This is soon changing!

With this new trend, IV fluids are now administered even in situations when they are not considered necessary. Most of the people who request for the IV fluids you will find them at home with the drip or at the office or better still at a hotel room.

There is a 'tour bus' that is mobile, offering to administer an IV hydration facility. Some of the services offered by this bus offer an IV hydration that comes with a mixture that is distinct of electrolytes and vitamins. Conditional to an individual's signs and budget, a pain medication, some anti-nausea medicine, a heartburn remedy and many other medications can be provided too.

This is a private service offered by private holders so it does not get catered for by your health insurance. In short it comes straight from your pocket and it's not cheap!

### *Reasons Why People May Wish for IVs*

Maybe there is an answer out there as to why people would diagnose themselves and buy IV fluids on a mobile bus. It still surprises why somebody would demand an IV on casual basis, but people are actually seeking to have them to cure hangovers, mild dehydration from flu or an over-exertion, jet lag, food poisoning, and even instant glow for hair and skin. Many people who can afford this service have just adopted it without questioning it.

IV fluids are incredibly necessary in cases that are genuine. For example, the very old and young who get flu do need the IV solution that comes from a hospital. Energetic individuals who carry enough strength around and can exercise a lot can ingest the fluids that the body needs.

IV fluids have now been marketed as improvements to how a person looks. This is all 'salesy' language to cause you to buy the IV fluids that you don't need. Beauty comes from a well-hydrated as well as properly nourished lifestyle.

It is important to emphasize that the situations that are causing the IV to be on high request are offered incorrectly. Jetlag and hangovers are not reasons enough to get an IV fluid. Orally drinking fluids is generally commended for hangover signs and jetlag.

Summing up, there is a sensible alternative to the IV solutions which is to orally ingest fluids. If you are capable of drinking lots of fluids, it is the easiest and preferable way to stay healthy. If you are too weak to drink orally and require rehydration, then you ought to seek treatment in a hospital. Before anything else, remember that the IV is invasive to your body and can cause serious infection to your body if the injection area becomes infected. A blood vessel can also become inflamed and clogged by some clot causing thrombosis.

These difficulties are not uncommon but it's not worth it to take risk with unnecessary treatments. Irrespective of how good the impression of an IV fluid at home is, it does not exceed the importance of drinking enough water at home in order to stay well hydrated. It is popular to see majority of people carrying their drinking water wherever they go with many working to consume at least 8 glasses every day. This is extremely necessary!

Then there are compelling stories about famous celebrities who describe how better they feel after getting an IV fluid treatment. Real stories that we listen to should come from those who were suffering greatly in the hospital bed not someone who is hanging a hangover for drinking the entire bar last night.

Scientists are yet to prove the advantages of IV fluids that are taken on demand. Though the medical dangers are low the financial costs are clearly high. The higher the amount of vitamins, electrolytes and medications in these drinks the crazier the costs.

Remember that these fluids can be attained in different ways by drinking fluids, obtaining self or pharmacy medications and taking vitamins of a generic nature for far less costs than the IV fluids.

In the 21st century, options have proven more accessible without necessarily getting medical exams or having a medical reason. You don't necessarily need a doctor to diagnose and prescribe rather you use MRI's, CT scans, Ultrasounds, genetic testing etc. to treat yourself.

Even though patient enablement is a wonderful thing, too much can become harmful. IV solutions on demand are not the finest example of patient empowerment. Such services are purely out to make money than help your health.

# Practice Questions

(1) If 0.00041kL of 0.9%NaCl IV needs to flow over a period of 1,074 minutes, calculate the rate of flow of the IV given the drop factor for the infusion set is 45gtts per milliliter. Give the flow rate of the IV in terms of gtts/min.

(2) The doctor has ordered infusion of 364,000 microLiters NS IV over a period of 354 minutes and this should be done via an infusion pump. Calculate the rate of IV flow in terms of milliliters per hour or mL/hr.

(3) The doctor has ordered the drug Metroprolol as found in the brand, Lopressor, and the dose is 9,000,000 micrograms or mcg PO. At the hospital the drug is available in tablet form, each weighing 0.003kg. Calculate the number of tablets the nurse needs to give the patient.

(4) The doctor orders the drug, Amoxicillin, and the dose is 7g. At the hospital pharmacy the drug is available in units of 12g for every 7mL. What amount is appropriate for the nurse to draw up?

(5) According to the doctor's order, a child weighing 25kg should be given fluid on a daily basis. What amount should the child receive each day measured in milliliters?

(6) The doctor orders fluids for a child who weighs 55lbs. What amount in milliliters should the nurse give this child each day?

(7) Find out the Sodium Chloride amount that is in 1.43 L NS.

(8) Calculate the flow rate of the IV in terms of mL/hr when an infant weighing just one kilogram needs to maintain the right fluid levels.

(9) The doctor's orders are to infuse 0.000047 kiloliters for a period of 20.1 hours using an infusion pump. What should the flow rate of the IV be in terms of milliliters per hour?

(10)    The medication record requires that you provide the patient with the drug, Dopamine, the dose being 12.6mg in 79mL and D5W, and to ensure infusion is done with the rate being 9,305mcg per hr. Find out the appropriate rate of flow in terms of mL per hr.

(11)    A patient is to receive through IV 299 milliliters of D5W over a period of 768 minutes. The drop factor for the infusion set is 66gtts per milliliter. Calculate the rate of IV flow, giving the answer in gtts/min.

(12)   A child weighs 16 kilograms, and the doctor has directed that this child receives an appropriate amount of fluid every day. How many milliliters of fluid should this child be given in one day?

(13)   The doctor orders the drug, Solumedrol, for a patient weighing 30 pounds, and the dosage is 1.5 milligrams per kilogram. At the hospital the drug is packaged as 75 milligrams per every 3 milliliters. What volume of the available medication should the nurse give the patient?

(14)   The medication order from the doctor read Amoxicillin 22,000 milligrams for the patient, but the hospital pharmacy had the drug dosage provided as 13 grams per 4 milliliters. Calculate how much medication the nurse is required to draw up.

(15)   The doctor has ordered the drug, Solumedrol, for a patient weighing 20 pounds, and the dosage is 1.5 milligrams per kilogram. At the hospital pharmacy the drug is available in a dosage of 75 milligrams per 2 milliliters. How much of the available medication, in terms of milliliters, is the nurse expected to administer?

(16)   The doctor orders a child who weighs 17 pounds to be given the drug, Solumedrol, and the dosage is 1.5 milligrams per kilogram. The Solumedrol medication at the nurse' disposal has its dosage as 75 milligrams per 3 milliliters. Calculate the number of milliliters the nurse should administer to the child.

(17)   Find out the quantity of sodium chloride present in 0.0006kL NS.

(18)   The doctor orders the drug, Solumedrol, to be administered to a child who weighs 43 pounds, and the dosage is 1.5 milligrams per kilogram. The drug the nurse has at her disposal has dosage in 75 milligrams per milliliter or mg/1mL. Calculate the amount of medication the nurse should administer to the child in milliliters (mL).

(19)   Find out the quantity of sodium chloride present in a volume, 0.00048 kiloliters, ½ NS.

(20)   From the medication record, the nurse can see the doctor has ordered the drug, Solumedrol, 2.5 milligrams per kilogram, for a child who weighs 27 kilograms. At the hospital pharmacy, the drug is available in dosage of 125 milligram per 2 milliliters. Calculate the number of milliliters the nurse should administer to the patient.

(21)   According to the medication order, the doctor ordered the drug, Solumedrol, for a child who weighed 14 kilograms, and the dosage was 2.5 milligrams per kilogram. At the medical facility, the drug available had a dosage of 125 milligrams per 3 milliliters. Calculate the number of milliliters of the available medication the nurse should administer to the child.

(22)    According to the medication order, a child whose weight is 13 pounds should be given the drug, Solumedrol, and the dosage is 1.5 milligrams per kilogram. However, the medical institution stocks this drug with its dosage being 75 milligrams per milliliter. Calculate the number of milliliters of the available medication the nurse should administer to the child.

(23)    According to the medication order, the patient is to receive the drug, Amoxicillin, and the dosage is 20 grams. The nurse find that the Amoxicillin at the hospital has dosage in 25 grams per 6 milliliters. How much of the available drug should the nurse on duty draw out to administer to the patient?

(24)    Find out the quantity of sodium chloride contained in 0.00058 kiloliters of Natural Saline (NS).

(25)    According the medication order, the patient should receive IV 0.00014 kiloliters or kL D5W using an infusion pump over a period of 5.2 hours. Calculate the flow rate of the IV in terms of milliliters per hour or mL/hr.

(26)    The doctor orders the drug, Solumedrol, for a child who weighs 3 kilograms. The dosage prescribed is 2.5 milligrams per kilogram, and the dosage of the medication available at the hospital is 125 milligrams per milliliter. Calculate the number of milliliters the nurse should administer to the patient.

(27)    According to the medication order, the patient should receive 0.015 kilograms of the drug Ampicillin. However, the medication available at the medical institution has its dosage in terms of 10,000 microgram tablets. How many tablets should the patient be given?

(28)    As per the medication record from the doctor, the patient needs to receive 17.5 milligrams of the drug, dopamine, which should be infused as 338 milliliters of D5W, and the rate of infusion should be 14,221 micrograms per hour (mcg/hr).

(29)    You have the infusion set with 25gtts/mL as the drop factor calibration, and you need to establish the rate of IV flow for an amount of 744 milliliters of Natural Saline (NS), which is supposed to be infused in a period of 14.6 hours. Give the answer for the rate of IV flow in terms of gtts/min.

(30)    There is a child at the hospital who weighs 27 kilograms and needs his fluid levels maintained. Calculate the ideal rate of IV flow in terms of milliliters per hour (mL/hr).

(31)    A child weighs 16 kilograms. What IV rate should be used in terms of milliliters per hour if the child is to maintain the appropriate level of fluids?

(32)   The doctor ordered that a patient weighing 36 kilograms be given aggrastat, and the dosage was 15.3 milligrams in 294 milliliters. The doctor also provided the rate of infusion via pump to be 10 micrograms per kilogram per hour. Calculate the rate of flow in terms of milliliters per hour.

(33)   A young person weighing 62 pounds requires a certain amount of fluid on a daily basis. How much fluid, in terms of milliliters, would you administer if this was your patient?

(34)   The medication order indicates the patient needs to receive 12 grams of Potassium Chloride, as in the brand, K-Dur, and the hospital has stocks of the drug in tablets of 12,000 milligrams each. How many tablets should the nurse administer to the patient?

(35)   The doctor orders a patient to be given 0.26 liters of NS through infusion over a period of 1,200 minutes. The drop factor calibration on the infusion set is 3gtts/mL. Calculate the rate of IV flow and give the answer in gtts/min.

(36)   The medication order shows a child who weighs 12 kilogram has been prescribed the drug, Solumedrol, and the dosage is 2.5 milligrams per kilogram. Meanwhile, the Solumedrol drug available at the hospital has dosage of 125 milligrams per 2 milliliters. Calculate the number of milliliters the nurse should administer to the patient.

(37)   The doctor ordered the patient to have 0.0003 kiloliters of 0.9% Sodium Chloride IV infused over a period of 10 hours. The drop factor for the infusion set is 79gtts per mL. Calculate the rate of flow of the IV and give the answer in gtts per minute.

(38)   Find out the quantity of Sodium Chloride contained in 0.2 liters NS.

(39)   According to the medication order, a patient needs to receive 514,000 microliters (mcL) NS IV through an infusion pump over a period of 1,368 minutes. Calculate the rate of IV flow in terms of milliliters per hour (mL/hr).

(40)   The doctor ordered that the patient receive 373 milliliters of IV infusion through an infusion pump over a period of 288 minutes. Calculate the rate of IV flow in terms of milliliters per hour (mL/hr).

(41)   The nurse is required to give the necessary level of fluids to a child who weighs 35 kilograms. How much, in milliliters, should the nurse give the child in one day?

(42)   The doctor orders an infant weighing one kilogram to be given the drug, Solumedro, and the dosage is 2.5 milligrams per kilogram. At the hospital pharmacy, the

Solumedrol available has dosage as 125 milligrams per 3 milliliters. Calculate the amount, in milliliters, the nurse should administer to the patient from what is available.

(43)   Find out the quantity of Sodium Chloride contained in 0.00056 kiloliters ¼ NS.

(44)   The doctor has ordered infusion of 379 milliliters NS IV by means of an infusion pump to a patient. Calculate the rate of IV in milliliters per hour (mL/hr).

(45)   According the medication record, the dosage ordered by the doctor to be infused over a period of 264 minutes is 0.76 liters D5W IV, and the fluid is to be administered using an infusion pump. Calculate the rate of IV flow in terms of milliliters per hour (mL/hr).

(46)   The doctor has ordered a child weighing 56 pounds be given sufficient fluids each day. How many milliliters would the nurse administer to the patient each day?

(47)   Find out the rate of IV flow when 142 milliliters of 0.9% Sodium Chloride (NaCl) are being infused over a period of 666 minutes. The drop factor for the infusion set is 97 gtts per milliliter (gtts/mL). Provide the answer in terms of gtts/min.

(48)   The doctor has ordered Solumedrol for a child whose weight is 25 pounds, and the dosage is 1.5 milligrams per kilogram. However, the dosage of the Solumedrol available at the hospital is 75 milligrams per milliliters (mg/mL). Calculate the amount of available drug the nurse needs to administer to the patient, and provide the answer in milliliters.

(49)   According to the medication record, the doctor has prescribed Potassium Chloride, as in the brand, K-Dur, and the dosage is 0.022 kilograms. The Potassium Chloride available in the pharmacy is packed in tablets of 23 grams each. Calculate the number of tablets that are supposed to be given to the patient.


(50)   Convert 40° Celsius to degrees Fahrenheit

Answer choices:

A.  88°F

B.  23°F

C.  104°F

D.  45°F

(51)    Convert 15° Celsius to degrees Fahrenheit.

Answer Choices:

   A. 59°F

   B. 29°F

   C. 108°F

   D. 30°F


(52)    Convert 52° Celsius to Fahrenheit

Answer Choices:

A.          25°F

B.          26°F

C.          104°F

D.          126°F


(53)    Convert 23.5° Celsius to Fahrenheit

Answer Choices:

A.          95°F

B.          74°F

C.          47°F

D.          235°F

(54)    Convert 32° Celsius to Fahrenheit

Answer Choices:

A.          90°F

B.          23°F

C.          -32°F

D.          64°F


(55)    Convert 100° Fahrenheit to Celsius

Answer Choices:

A.          50°C

B.          32°C

C.          38°C

D.          200°C


(56)    Convert 55° Fahrenheit to Celsius

Answer Choices:

A.          28°C

B.          36°C

C.          23°C

D.          13° C

(57)   Convert 60° Fahrenheit to Celsius

Answer Choices:

A.            -60°C

B.            120°C

C.            16°C

D.            -30° C

(58)   Convert 39° Fahrenheit to Celsius

A.  -60°C

B.  4°C

C.  93°C

D.  -39° C

(59)   Convert 78° Fahrenheit to Celsius

A.  26°C

B.  39°C

C.  -78°C

D.  87° C

(60)  Which Arabic number is written as LXXVII using Roman numerals?

Answer Choices:

A   57

B   77

C   27

D   527

(61)  What is the amount represented by the numeral written in Roman as IVss?

Answer Choices:

A. 6 1/2

B. 4

C. 4 ½

D. 15

(62)  State the number of times within a period of 24 hours a nurse needs to administer medication to a patient if the medication order reads 'gtt II o.s. tid'.

Answer Choices:

A. Three

B. Eleven

C. Once

D. Two

(63)  Provide the value of X as used in the equation, 3X = 51.

Answer Choices:

A. 51

B. 3

C. 17

D. 4

(64)  Calculate the value of X in the equation, ½ X = 5mg

Answer Choices:

A. 1mg

B. 10mg

C. 0.5mg

D. 5.5mg

(65)  Calculate the value of X in the equation, 0.5x + 1 = 2

Answer Choices:

A. 0.10

B. 1.5

C. 1/2

D. 2

(66)   Calculate the value of X in the equation, 2.5mg = ¼ X

Answer Choices:

A. 2.5

B. 10mg

C. 10

D. 10mcg

(67)   Calculate the appropriate amount of Promethazine Hydrochloride injection, in milliliters, the nurse would administer to the patient if the doctor prescribed 12.5mg of the drug and the drug at the hospital had dosage of 25mg/mL.

Answer Choices:

A. 0.5mL

B. 25mL

C. 37.5mL

D. 6.25mL

(68)   Calculate the number of grams of the drug, Thiabendazole, contained in an oral suspension bottle of the drug whose size is 120mL if the dosage label indicates 500mg/5cc.

Answer Choices:

A. 100g

B. 0.01g

C. 12g

D. 1,200g

(69)   Calculate the number of milligrams in 0.5 grams.

Answer Choices:

A.  500mg.

B.  5mg.

C.  5,000mg.

D.  0.0005mg.

(70)   Calculate the number of liters made up of 27.3 milliliters.

Answer Choices:

A.  2,730L

B.  0.273L

C.  0.0273L

D.  27,300L

(71)   Calculate generally the number of fluid ounces comprising eight fluid ounces.

Answer Choices:

A.  240mL.

B.  128mL.

C.  120mL.

D.  3.75mL.

(72)   Calculate the number of milliliters that make up 3 US pints.

Answer Choices

A.  1,950 mL

B.  90mL

C.  1,419 mL

D.  195 mL


(73)   The hospital pharmacy has the injection drug, Chlordiazepoxide hydrochloride, as in the brand, Librium, which is supplied in dry powder form. The medication comes in packets of 100mg, accompanied by a separate vial of 2mL diluent. Find out how many such vials should be opened in order to dilute a dose of 30mg of the drug.

Answer Choices:

A.  13.5mL

B.  0.6mL

C.  0.6mL

D.  3.3mL


(74)   How many milliliters (mL) are there in 9 ounces (oz)?

Answer choices:

A.  0.3mL

B.  2.7mL

C.  270mL

D.  0.27mL

(75)    How many micrograms (mcg) are there in 27 milligrams (mg)?

Answer Choices:

A.  370mcg

B.  2,700mcg

C.  27,000mcg

D.  0.0027mcg


(76)    How many ounces (oz)  are there in 15 milliliters (mL)?

Answer Choices:

A.  15 ounces

B.  ½ ounce

C.  30 ounces

D.  2 ounces


(77)    How many milligrams (mg) are there in 956 micrograms (mcg)?

Answer Choices:

A.  96mg

B.  9,560mg

C.  0.0096mg

D.  0.96mg

(78)    Calculate the number of ounces (oz) in 29 ½ milliliters (mL) of liquid.

Answer Choices:

A.  29.5 ounces

B.  885 ounces

C.  0.98 ounces

D.  30 ounces


(79)    How many milliliters (mL) are there in 10 cubic centimeters (cc)?

Answer Choices:

A.  2.5 milliliters

B.  10 milliliters

C.  0.5 milliliters

D.  None of the choices provided


(80)    Calculate the number of milliliters (mL) in 5.25 ounces (oz).

Answer Choices:

A.  6 milliliters

B.  3.5 milliliters

C.  157.5 milliliters

D.  5 milliliters

(81)    How many cc are there in 35mL?

Answer Choices:

A.  350 cc

B.  3,500 cc

C.  17.5 cc

D.  35 cc

(82)    How many milliliters (mL) are there in 7 teaspoons (tsp)?

Answer Choices:

A.  35 milliliters

B.  7 milliliters

C.  0.7 milliliters

D.  5 milliliters

(83)    How man milliliters are there in 5 liters?

Answer Choices:

A.  5 milliliters

B.  5,000 milliliters

C.  0.005 milliliters

D.  50 milliliters

(84)   How many teaspoons are made up of 55 milliliters?

Answer Choices:

A.  275 teaspoons

B.  11 teaspoons

C.  5.5 teaspoons

D.  0.55 teaspoons

(85)   How many liters comprise 19 milliliters?

Answer Choices:

A.  0.019 liters

B.  19,000 liters

C.  190 liters

D.  1.9 liters

(86)   Calculate the number of milligrams that comprise 4 ½ grams.

Answer Choices:

A.  4,500 milligrams

B.  4.5 milligrams

C.  0.045 milligrams

D.  7 milligrams

(87)  How many grams are made up of 1,200 micrograms?

Answer Choices:

A.  1.2 grams

B.  1,200 grams

C.  0.0012 grams

D.  12 grams

(88)  How many mcg make 9g?

Answer Choices:

A.  90 mcg

B.  9,000 mcg

C.  0.009 mcg

D.  9,000,000 mcg

(89)  How many grams comprise 68 micrograms?

Answer Choices:

A.  0.000068 grams

B.  68,000 grams

C.  0.0068 grams

D.  14 grams

(90)   How many milliliters are in 6 teaspoons?

Answer Choices:

A.  30 milliliters

B.  1/6 milliliters

C.  0.6 milliliters

D.  5 milliliters

(91)   How many liters are there in 9 teaspoons?

Answer Choices:

A.  0.009 liters

B.  45 liters

C.  0.045 liters

D.  450 liters

(92)   Calculate the number of cc in 12L.

Answer Choices:

A.  0.012 L

B.  12,000 cc

C.  5,000 cc

D.  12 cc

(93)  How many ounces (oz) are there in 16 milliliters (mL)?

Answer Choices:

A. 16000 ounces

B. 0.54 ounces

C. 0.16 ounces

D. 530 ounces

(94)  Calculate the number of kilograms comprising 250 pounds.

Answer Choices:

A. 113.6 kilograms

B. 550 kilograms

C. 0.025 kilograms

D. 2.5 kilograms

(95)  Calculate the number of pounds contained in 195 kilograms.

Answer Choices:

A. 429 pounds

B. 195,000 pounds

C. 0.0195 pounds

D. 88.64 pounds

(96)   Calculate the number of milligrams comprising 9 micrograms.

Answer Choices:

A.  0.009 milligrams

B.  9,000 milligrams

C.  0.001 milligrams

D.  9 milligrams


(97)   Calculate the number of milliliters contained in 26 ounces.

Answer Choices:

A.  26,000 milliliters

B.  769 milliliters

C.  0.769 milliliters

D.  13 milliliters


(98)   Find out the number of liters that comprise 360 milliliters.

Answer Choices:

A.  36,000 liters

B.  720 liters

C.  0.36 liters

D.  0.0027 liters

(99)   In this question you are required to find out how much Amoxicillin a nurse needs to draw up in order to have 23000 mg of Amoxicillin, bearing in mind that Amoxicillin is available as 1,000,000 mcg per 9ml.

(100)   This question requires you to calculate the flow rate in mL/hr, where a patient is to be given 18.8 mg of dopamine which is available in 363 mL of D5W which is to be infused at the rate of 13,175 mcg / hr.

(101)   In this question we are required to find out how many mL of Solumedrol a nurse should administer to a child who weighs 29 kg, if Solumedrol is available as 125mg/ 3 ml and it was ordered as 2.5 mg/kg.

(102)   In this question you are required to calculate the number of tablets a nurse should administer in order to achieve 9,000,000 mcg of Ampicillin, if Ampicillin is available as 20g tablets.

(103)   In this question you are required to calculate the amount of Solumedrolto be administered to a child who weighs 14 lb, if the doctor ordered 1.5 mg/kg and Solumedrol is available as 75 mg/ 1 mL.

(104)   In this question you are needed to calculate the amount of Sodium chloride in 1.5 L ½ NS.

(105)   Find out the quantity of sodium chloride contained in 1.5 liters 1/2 NS.

(106)   The doctor has written a medication order for a child who weighs 15 pounds (lb). Calculate the rate of IV in terms of milliliters per hr (mL/hr) in order to ensure the right fluid level is maintained.

(107)   A medical practitioner has ordered that a child weighing 13 pounds be given the right amount of fluid each day. Calculate the appropriate amount in milliliters?

(108)   The doctor ordered 0.00077 kiloliters (kL) D5W IV to be infused in a span of 15.6 hours using an infusion pump. Calculate the rate of IV flow in terms of milliliters per hour (mL/hr).

(109)   A young girl in the ward weighs 38 kilograms and the doctor has ordered that she be given enough fluid each day via IV. What should be the rate of IV flow in terms of milliliters per hour (mL/hr)?

(110)   The medical practitioner has ordered Potassium Chloride, as in the brand, K-Dur, and the amount in the order is 10,000,000 micrograms. However, from the hospital

pharmacy, only 2 gram tablets are available. Calculate the number of tablets to be dispensed to the patient.

(111)   The medical practitioner has ordered the drug, Solumedrol, 2.5 milligram per kilogram (mg/kg) and the prescription is for an infant who weighs just a kilogram, Considering the drug available at the pharmacy is in 125 milligrams per 2 milliliters (mg/ml), calculate the amount of fluid the nurse must administer to the infant.

(112)   The doctor has ordered 22 grams of Potassium Chloride, as in brand K-Dur, but the drug available is in tablets of 23,000,000 micrograms. How many of those tablets is the nurse supposed to dispense to the patient?

(113)   The doctor has prescribed Amoxicillin suspension for a one year old child who weighs 22 pound. The dosage for this child who has otitis media is 40 milligrams per kilogram per day, and it is divided BID. The hospital medication is packaged in concentrations of 400 milligrams per 5 milliliters.

Find out the Amoxicillin dose in terms of milliliters.

(114)   The medical practitioner has prescribed ceftriaxone for a child whose weight is 18 kilograms. This dose, which is meant to treat meningitis, is 100 milligram per kilogram per day, and it is to be administered in IV. The drug comes to the hospital pre-diluted, and it is in a concentration of 40 milligrams per milliliter.

Calculate the dosage the nurse is supposed to administer in milliliters.

(115)   In this question, you are required to calculate the flow rate in mL/hr in which you are going to set an IV pump in order to administer a bolus dose of 60 units / kg to a patient who weighs 198 lbs. The doctor orders that the Heparin IV drip starts at 16units/kg and you are offered with a Heparin bag that reads 12,500 units/ 250mL.

(116)   In this question we are required to find out the number of units a patient is receiving per hour if the Heparin drip is running at 36 mL/hr and the Heparin bag reads 12,500 units/ 250 mL.

(117)   In this question we are tasked with calculating the amount of Heparin a patient receives per hour if the Heparin drip is running at 29 mL/hr and the Heparin bag reads 10,000 units/ 100 mL.

(118)   We are required to calculate the flow rate in mL/hr, for a patient who weighs 129 lbs. The drip starts at 24 units/kgs/hr and the Heparin bags reads 25,000 units/250 Ml.

(119)   The medication order indicates the patient, who is a boy with leukemia aged 4yrs, requires the drug, vincristine. The boy weighs 37 pounds and happens to be 97

centimeters in height. The order indicates a dose of 2 milligrams per square meter but the drug at the hospital is in dosage of 1 milligram per milliliter.

Find out the vincristine dose to be dispensed in milliliters.

(120) The doctor has prescribed 4 tablets of the medication, Z, and the patient is to take it two times a day, 6/7. How many should the nurse dispense to the patient for the full dose?

(121) The physician has prescribed a patient 15 milliliters of cough medication, to take 4 times each day for seven days. How many doses should the patient be given?

# Answers to Practice Questions

(1) This question required that you calculate the rate of IV flow in gtts/min.

The answer to this question is <u>17gtts/min</u>

In providing answers to such questions involving volume, time and drop rate, the units are very important and you should ensure the units you provide to your correct values are also the appropriate ones.

<u>Workings</u>

The correct formula to use is:

Volume in milliliters / Time in minutes x Drop factor in gtts/mL = Appropriate Rate of Flow in gtts/min

First of all you need to convert the units of volume given in kiloliters to milliliters, and to do this you need to multiply them by 1,000 to get volume in liters and then multiply those units further by 1,000 to get the volume in milliliters.

0.00041kL x 1,000 = 0.41L

0.41L x 1,000 = 410mL

You now have the right units to calculate the rate of IV flow in gtts/min.

410mL / 1,074min x 45gtts/mL

If you multiply across first, what you get is:

(410mL x 45gtts) / 1,074 min x 1/1mL

This works to 18,450gtts/1,074min because the ml units will have cancelled each other out both above and below. After doing your calculation you will have:

17.178gtts/min, but since drops are only given in full when it comes to medication dosage, the correct answer is 17gtts/min.

(2) The question required that you calculate the rate of IV flow in terms of mL/hr.

The correct answer is 61.7mL / hr.

Workings

The first step you need to do is identify the formula relevant to this kind of problem. In this case the relevant formula is:

Volume in Milliliters / Time in Hours = Appropriate Rate of Flow in mL/hr

Since the time element in the formula is given in hours, you need to convert the 354 minutes indicated by the doctor to hours. To change minutes to hours you need to divide the value you have by 60.

354 minutes ÷ 60 = 5.9 hours

Also, the doctor has ordered the fluid to be given in units of mcL yet the formula uses fluid units in mL. So you need to convert the microliters to milliliters. The way to do this is to divide the units ordered by 1,000.

So the rate of IV flow required is 364 milliliters per 5.9 hours, which can be simplified by calculating:

364mL / 5.9hr = 61.69 or 61.7 mL / hr

(3) The question required that you calculate the number of tablets the nurse should give the patient.

The correct answer is 3 tablets.

This kind of calculation deals with mass versus mass, where the doctor's prescription is in mass and you need to gauge it against another mass. The appropriate formula to use to solve this problem is:

Mass ordered / Mass available = Number of tablets needed

Begin by converting the mass of tablets available from kilograms to micrograms so you can have like terms and units that are easy to work with.

0.003kg x 1,000 = 3 grams

3g x 1,000 = 3,000milligrams

3,000mg x 1,000 = 3,000,000 micrograms

Now following the formula, Mass ordered / Mass available = Number of tablets needed:

9,000,000 / 3,000,000= Number of tablets needed

9,000,000 ÷ 3,000,000 = 3 tablets

(4) This question required that you calculate the amount of Amoxicillin the nurse ought to draw up when the drug at the hospital is in 12g/7mL.

The right answer is 4.1mL

<u>Workings</u>

The formula suitable for use when trying to solve such a problem is:

Amount ordered / Amount available x Volume in the Available Quantity = Amount of Liquid Needed

In this case, you need to calculate 7g / 12g x 7mL

First of all, the units of grams/g above and below will cancel out completely, and now you can proceed to calculate:

7/12 x 7mL

7 x 7mL = 49mL, and when you divide this by 12 you get 4.08mL, which you can round up to 4.1mL.

(5) This question required that you calculate the fluid amount to give an infant weighing 25kg each day, in milliliters per day.

The right answer is 1,600mL.

Workings

To solve this problem you need to have understood the topic on fluid maintenance. There is a schedule that helps you identify the fluid level to give a patient based on the patient's body weight.

Since a child weighing between 20kg and 70kg needs to receive 1,500mL each day and in addition to this another 20mL for every kilogram above the 20kg level, you need to first calculate the number of kilograms the child weighs above 20kg.

25kg − 20kg = 5kg

Up to the 20kg mark, you need to give the child 1,500mL.

For the 5kg above the 20kg mark, you need to give 5 x 20mL, which is 100mL.

Adding the two amounts, 1,500mL + 100mL you get 1,600mL.

(6) This question demanded that you calculate the amount of fluid in milliliters the nurse should give a child weighing 55lbs each day.

The right answer is 1,600mL.

Workings

This question seeks to establish if you understand matters of fluid maintenance particularly when the patient's weight is given in units that vary from the ones used in the schedule of weights versus units of fluid.

The first thing you ought to do is convert the child's weight given in lbs to kilograms, and to do this you need to divide the value that is in lbs by 2.2.

55 pounds x 2.2 = 25 kilograms

So, basically, this question is similar to the previous one with the difference being in this one the weight is given in pounds and not in kilograms as in the previous one.

As in the previous problem, you need to remember the range of weights within which 25kg falls, and this is between 20kg and 70kg.

You also need to remember what it says about the weights within this range, and that is for the first 20kg you give the patient 1,500mL of fluid. Then for every kilogram over and above this level you multiply by 20mL.

So your calculations here should be 1,500mL + (5 x 20)mL = 1,500mL + 100mL

The right answer is 1,600mL.

(7) This question required that you find out the Sodium Chloride amount that is in 1.43L NS.

The right answer is 12.9g.

A question like this one seeks to find out if you understand how to calculate the level of concentration in a given amount of IV fluid.

The first thing you ought to remember is that NS is always 0.9% NaCl, where NaCl stands for Sodium Chloride. Then remember the right formula to use, which is:

Percentage of Concentration / 100 x Volume in milliliters = Dosage required in grams

As you can see, the formula deals with milliliters while the question gives the volume in liters. So you need to convert the units given in liters to milliliters. To convert liters to milliliters you need to multiply the units you have by 1,000, so in this case:

1.43 liters x 1,000 = 1,430 milliliters

Now using the identified formula:

0.9 / 100 x 1,430 milliliters = Sodium Chloride amount in grams

0.9/100 x 1,430 milliliters = 1,287ml/100, whose outcome is 12.87g. This can be rounded upwards to become 12.9g.

(8) This question required that you calculate the flow rate of the IV in terms of mL/hr when an infant weighing just one kilogram had to maintain the appropriate fluid levels.

The right answer is 4.17mL per hr.

Workings

This is another problem where you need to remember the schedule of fluid maintenance according to body weight. For an infant weighing 1kg, its fluid level would fall in the range of weights between below a kilogram to 10 kilograms. Children whose weight falls within this range require fluids of 100mL for every kilogram they weigh.

Hence in this case, you would be required to multiply 100mL by 1 to get the amount of fluid to give the infant.

100mL x 1 = 100mL

You have accomplished the first step of establishing the volume of fluid the infant needs. The next step will be to calculate the flow rate of the IV given the volume in mL.

The way to handle this stage of the question is to consider the volume of liquid, which is 100mL, and the time under consideration, which is a single day. The appropriate formula for IV rate calculation under the circumstances is:

Volume of fluid in ml / Time in hours = Rate of IV Flow in mL/hr

You know the fluid the infant needs, which is 100mL, and obviously, there are 24 hours comprising a day. Your calculations should, therefore, look like this:

100ml/24hr = Rate of IV Flow in mL/hr

Once you solve this calculation you find the rate of flow to be 4.1666, which can be rounded upwards to 4.17mL/hr.

(9) This question required that you calculate the flow rate of the IV given the volume of fluid and the period over which to infuse it, and the answer should be in mL per hr.

The right answer is 2.3mL per hr.

The most appropriate formula to use when doing calculations involving volume, time and flow rate is:

Volume in Milliliters / Time in Hours = Rate of flow in Milliliters per Hour

Since the volume is to be given in milliliters and the formula still uses milliliters for the volume, you need to first of all convert the volume provided in the question in kiloliters to milliliters.

0.000047kL x 1,000 = 0.04

7L

0.047L x 1,000 = 47mL

Now back to the formula:

Volume in Milliliters / Time in Hours = Rate of flow in Milliliters per Hour

47ml/20.1 hr gives 2.338mL/hr, which can be rounded to 2.3mL/hr.

(10)    In this question you were supposed to calculate the appropriate rate of flow in terms of mL per hr, having been provided with the volume and medication mass as well as the concentration of Dextrose.

The right answer is 58.3 milliliters per hour (mL/hr)

Here you need to remember the formula used where the terms to work with are the mass, time as well as the rate of IV flow. The most suitable here is:

Amount ordered per hour / Amount available x Volume of fluid = Rate of IV flow in mL/hr


Workings

Since you need to work with like terms, begin by converting the amount in mcg to mg. To convert 9,305 micrograms to grams you need to divide the amount by 1,000.

9,305mcg ÷ 1,000 = 9.305g

Now, applying the formula, Amount ordered per hour / Amount available x Volume of fluid:

9.305 milligrams per hour / 12.5 milligrams  x 79 milliliters

First of all, you can get rid of the milligram units by canceling the one accompanying the numerator against the one accompanying the denominator. Next, multiply the figures across:

 (9.305 per hour x 79 milliliters) / 12.6 = 735.095 milliliters per hour / 12.6

The result of the division is 58.3408, which can be rounded to 58.3 milliliters per hour (mL/hr).

(11)    This question required that you calculate the rate of IV flow given the volume to be dispensed and the time over which the infusion will take place, and giving the answer in gtts/min.

The right answer is 26gtts per minute (gtts/min)

The most helpful formula in this situation is:

Volume in milliliters / Time in minutes x Drop Factor in gtts per milliliter = Rate of Flow in gtts/min

When you put in the actual values, your calculation will look like this:

(299 milliliters / 768 minutes) x 66 gtts per milliliter

You can begin by dividing diagonally, where 66 divided by 6 gives you 11 and 768 divided by 6 gives you 128. Your work will now look like this:

(299 milliliters / 128 minutes) x 11 gtts per milliliter

Multiply across, 299 x 11 and you will get 3,289, and when you divide that by 128 you get 25.69. The units remain as they are, and milliliters over minutes provide the rate while the gtts is the unit of the drops. Because drops can only come in whole numbers, your answer must be 26gtts/min.

(12)   This question required that you calculate the daily fluid amount to give a child weighing 16kg.

The right answer is 1,300mL.

Workings

You need to recognize this question as one associated with maintenance of fluids in the body, and this will straightaway take you to the schedule of weights versus suitable amounts of fluids per day.

For a child who weighs anywhere from 10 kilograms to 20 kilograms, their daily fluid intake should be first of all 1,000 milliliters, and for every kilogram over and above 10 kilograms the child should receive 50 milliliters.

For this particular question, there are 6 kilograms above the basic 10 kilograms, and so your workings ought to look like this:

1,000mL + (6 x 50mL) = 1,000mL + 300mL = 1,300mL

So each day this 16kg weighing child should receive 1,300mL of fluids.

(13)   This question required that you calculate the number of milliliters to be administered to a patient whose weight is 30 pounds, given the recommended amount of drug per one kilogram of the patient's weight.

The right answer is 0.82 milliliters (mL)

<u>Workings</u>

You must recognize this question as one dealing with dosage ordered according to the patient's weight, and once you do so, you realize the way to find out the right amount required to be dispensed is the patient's weight multiplied by the right dosage per kilogram.

At this juncture you will see the need to convert the units of the patient's weight as given, because it is in pounds yet the suitable formula uses kilograms. To convert 30 pounds to kilograms you simply calculate:

30 pounds ÷ 2.2 = 13.63636 kilograms or 13.6364kg

First of all, the drug dosage to give is:

13.6364 x 1.5mg = 20.4546mg

From this point onward, you need to be thinking in terms of mass per liquid amount so as to identify the appropriate formula to provide the answer needed. Remember the available medication is in 75mg per 3mL. Use the formula:

(Amount ordered / Amount available) x Volume in the Available = Appropriate number of milliliters

So you proceed to work as follows:

(20.4545 milligrams / 75 milligrams) x 3 milliliters

The units of milligrams above and below cancel out completely, and when you do a diagonal division, 3 divided by 3 you get 1 while 75 divided by 3 gives you 25. So now you have:

20.4545/25 x 1 milliliter = (0.81818/1) x 1 milliliter

Multiply the numbers across and you get 0.81818 milliliters, which can be rounded to 0.82 milliliters (mL).

(14)    In this question you are required to calculate the amount of medication the nurse is supposed to draw up from the one available, considering the doctor has prescribed the medication in milligrams and the one available is in grams per given volume.

The right answer for this question is 6.8mL

To answer this question properly, you need to have understood the dosage calculations topic on mass as a proportion of liquid. Here the order is in milligrams and what is available is in grams, so there will also be some conversion involved. The most suitable formula to use in solving this problem is:

Amount ordered / Amount available x Volume per Amount Available = Liquid amount needed

Begin by converting 13 grams to milligrams, and you will achieve this by multiplying that amount of medication available by 1,000.

13 grams x 1,000 = 13,000 milligrams

Now the chosen formula can work as illustrated here below:

22,000 milligrams / 13,000 milligrams x 4 milliliters

First of all, the milligram units above and below will cancel out completely. Then you can proceed to divide 22,000 by 13,000 and you will get 1.69, whereas the denominator will now be 1. In short, you now have:

1.69/1 x 4 milliliters

Since whatever number you put over 1 remains as itself, you can conclude that what you have is:

1.69 x 4 milliliters, which produces 6.76 milliliters (mL), and this can be aptly rounded upwards to become 6.8mL.

(15)    In this question, you were required to calculate the amount of medication the nurse needed to get from that available at the hospital, to administer to the patient.

The right answer is 0.36 milliliters (mL)

<u>Workings</u>

This question is testing your understanding of how dosage is calculated when given the patient's weight and varying medication units. The appropriate formula to apply here is:

Patient's weight in kilograms x Dosage per kilogram = Dosage to Administer

You will notice that while the doctor has given the dosage in mg per kg, the child's weight has been recorded in pounds. So it is imperative that you convert the child's weight into kilograms as well. To change pounds into kilograms you just divide the weight figure by 2.2 as follows:

20 pounds ÷ 2.2 = 9.0909 kilograms

Now, following the chosen formula you can work as follows:

Patient's weight in kilograms x Dosage per kilogram = Drug to Administer

9.0909 kilograms x 1.5 milligrams per kilogram = Drug to administer

9.0909 kilograms /1 x 15 milligrams / 1 kilogram

You can cancel the kilogram units diagonally, and again any number over 1 is just the number itself, so you will remain with:

9.0909 x 1.5 milligrams

After doing the multiplication you will have 13.63635 milligrams, which is the amount of drug the doctor prescribed.

However, the drug at the nurse' disposal is measured in 75mg per 2mL, so you must perform further calculations to establish the exact amount of the medication at the hospital the nurse should administer to the patient.

The appropriate formula here is:

Amount ordered / Amount available x Volume for the Drug Available = Volume of Medication Needed

13.6364 milligrams / 75 milligrams x 2 milliliters

You can begin by canceling out the milligram units, above and below.

Next, multiply the figures across and divide the result by 75. The next step will look like this:

(13.6364 x 2 milliliters) / 75 = 0.3636mL or simply 0.36mL

(16)    This question required that you calculate the amount of medication the nurse should administer to the child in milliliters, or the dosage in milliliters, where the doctor's order provides the prescription in terms of milligrams per a kilogram of the child's weight.

The right answer is 0.46 milliliters

<u>Workings</u>

If you understood the calculations on dosage when given in terms of the patient's weight, then you will know the best formula to use here is:

Weight of Patient in Kilograms x Dosage given per kilogram = Needed Dosage

You will also notice that there is need to convert units of weight so that the units in the dosage match the units of the patient's weight. In this case you need to convert the patient's 17 pounds to kilograms, and to do this you divide the number of pounds by 2.2.

17 pounds ÷ 2.2 = 7.72727 kilograms

Now using the identified formula:

Weight of Patient in Kilograms x Dosage given per kilogram = Needed Dosage

7.72727 kilograms x 1.5 milligrams / 1 kilogram = Needed Dosage

You can cancel the kilogram units diagonally, and then multiply 7.72727 by 1.5 milligrams.

7.7272 x 1.5 milligrams = 11.5909 milligrams

Having established the medication the child requires, you now need to calculate how much of the available medication the child ought to receive in order to have the Solumedrol amount of 11.5909 milligrams. The medication available has dosage in terms of 75 milligrams per 3 milliliters.

This is an issue of mass versus liquid, and the appropriate formula is:

(Medication ordered / Medication Available) x Volume per Medication Available = Milliliters Needed

(11.5909 milligrams / 75 milligrams) x 3 milliliters = Milliliters Needed

You can begin by canceling out the 3 against the 75 beneath, so that you now have:

(11.5909 milligrams / 25 milligrams) x 1 milliliter = Milliliters Needed

Next you can cancel out the milligram units above and below, and when you solve the rest of the fraction you will have:

0.46363 milliliters, which you can simply write as 0.46 milliliters (mL)

(17)    In this question, the requirement was that you find out the quantity of sodium chloride present in 0.0006kL NS.

The right answer for this question is 5.4 grams (g)

Workings

This question demands that you remember how to calculate amounts in IV fluids or the fluid's concentration.

As you prepare to find out the quantity of sodium chloride present in 0.0006kL NS, it is important to remember that NS is always 0.9% sodium chloride (NaCl). The appropriate formula for this calculation is:

(Percentage of Concentration / 100) x Volume in milliliters = Dosage quantity in grams (g)

However, there is need to first convert kiloliters to milliliters, so that you will be working with like terms. To convert kL to mL you need to multiply the value you have by 1,000 to first get the value in L, and then by 1,000 to get the value in mL. So here you will calculate:

0.0006 kiloliters x 1,000 = 0.6L

0.6 liters x 1,000 = 600 milliliters

The formula you identified can now work to give you the quantity of sodium chloride in the amount of liquid provided.

0.9%/100 x 600

You can begin by canceling out the denominator against 600, and you will remain with:

0.9% of 600 or 0.9 x 100/100 x 600

The denominator cancels vertically with the other 100 that is the numerator, and so you remain with:

0.9 x 600

This works out to 5.400, or simply 5.4 grams (g)

(18)    This question required that you calculate the amount of the drug, Solumedrol, in milliliters the nurse should administer to a child whose weight is 43 pounds.

The right answer for this question is 0.39 milliliters (mL)

<u>Workings</u>

This question that tests how well you can calculate dosage when given the patient's weight and the dosage available in varying units, requires that you use the formula:

Patient's weight in Kilograms x Dosage per Kilogram = Dosage needed

However, the first step ought to be conversion of the child's weight from pounds to kilograms, and to do this you need to divide it by 2.2.

43 pounds ÷ 2.2 = 19.5454 kilograms

Now back to the formula for dosage:

19.5454 kilograms x 1.5 milligrams per kilogram works out as:

(19.5454 kilograms x 1.5 milligrams) / 1 kilogram

When the kilogram units above and below cancel out, you are left with:

19.5454 x 1.5 milligrams, which works out to 29.31818 milligrams

From here henceforth you will be working to solve a problem of mass versus liquid, and the appropriate formula is:

Amount ordered / Amount available x Volume for the Drug Available = Liquid Needed

(29.3182 milligrams / 75 milligrams) x 1 milliliter

The milligram units with both the numerator and denominator cancel out, so that you have:

29.3182/75 x 1 milliliter

The calculations here result to 0.3909 milliliters, which can be written as 0.39 milliliters (mL)

(19)    In this question, you were required to find out the sodium chloride quantity present in 0.00048 kiloliters ½ NS.

Then answer for this question is 2.2 grams (g)

<u>Workings</u>

Here you are being tested in whether you can calculate amounts of mass in a given amount of IV fluid. First of all you need to keep in mind that NS always has 0.9% sodium chloride (NaCl), and so when it comes to the units given in the question:

0.9% x ½ = 0.45%

The formula to use here is:

Percentage of Concentration / 100 x Volume in milliliters = Amount of Dosage in grams

Begin by converting 0.00048 kiloliters to milliliters, and you can do this through two stages, one converting the kiloliters to liters and then the liters to milliliters. In each of the stages, you need to multiply the value you have by 1,000.

0.00048 kiloliters x 1,000 = 0.48 liters

0.48 liters x 1,000 = 480 milliliters

Now using the formula you identified:

0.45% x 480 milliliters

This is the same as:

0.45 x (100/100 x 1/100) x 480 milliliters

After the denominator, 100, cancels out with the 100 that is the numerator, you are left with 0.45 x 1/100 x 480 milliliters, which produces 2.16g or 2.2g.

(20)  This question required that you calculate the number of milliliters the nurse should administer to the patient.

The right answer is 1.08 milliliters (mL)

<u>Workings</u>

You are capable of making the correct calculations here once you have mastered how to calculate dosage that is given in terms of patient's weight. The appropriate formula to use here is:

Weight in terms of Kilograms x Dosage in terms of Kilograms = Dosage Needed

In this particular question, the units of weight are similar, both in the dosage and for the child, so no weight conversions are required before applying the dosage formula.

27 kilograms x 2.5 milligrams per kilogram can be expressed as:

27 kilograms x 2.5 milligrams / 1 kilogram

The kilogram units can then cancel out, and you will be left with:

27 x 2.5 milligrams, and this works out to 67.5 milligrams (mg)

Having established the dosage the child needs in milliliters, you now need to find out the amount of available medication the nurse ought to administer in milliliters. In short, the doctor has ordered that the child receives 67.5 milligrams of medication, yet what the hospital provides has dosage of 125 milligrams for every 2 milliliters. The appropriate formula to use is:

Medication ordered / Medication available x Volume per Medication Available = Milliliters Needed

67.5 milligrams / 125 milligrams x 2 milliliters = Milliliters Needed

The milligram units can cancel out completely, above and below, and then you can proceed with the multiplication.

67.5 x 2 milliliters = 135 milliliters

125 x 1 = 125

So now what you have is 135 milliliters / 125

And the answer is 1.08 milliliters (mL)

(21)   This question required that you calculate the number of milliliters the nurse needed to administer to the child who weighed 14 kilogram.

The right answer is 0.84 milliliters.

Once you have mastered how to calculate dosage based on the patient's body weight you cannot have a problem solving a question like this, and it is important that you give your answer in the units required.

The formula to help you make the necessary calculations is:

Patient's weight in Kilograms x Dosage per Kilogram = Needed Dosage

Since the patient in this case weighs 14 kilograms and the dosage ordered by the doctor is 2.5 milligrams per kilogram, the required dosage for the patient should be:

14 kilogram x 2.5 milligrams per kilogram. This can be expressed as:

(14 kilogram x 2.5 milligrams) / 1 kilogram

The kilogram units above and below cancel out to leave 14 x 2.5 milligrams that works out to become 35 milligrams.

Looking back at the question, you can see it requires that you provide the answer as the amount of medication from what is available at the hospital the nurse ought to give the patient, and the answer needs to be in milliliters. Clearly here it is a matter of working with mass versus liquid.

In this case the doctor has ordered 35 milligrams but the hospital avails the medication in terms of 125 milligrams per 3 milliliters. The formula that is helpful in such cases is:

Medication ordered / Medication available  x Volume per Medication Available = Milliliters Needed

35 milligrams / 125 milligrams x 3 milliliters

The milligram units above and below cancel out completely, and if you divide 35 by 5 and 125 by 5 you get:

7/25 x 3 milliliters, which works to become 21/25 milliliters or 0.84 milliliters (mL)

(22)  This question required that you calculate the number of milliliters to be given a child who weighs 13 pounds when the doctor has ordered Solumedrol with the dosage being 1.5 milligram per kilogram.

The right answer is 0.12 milliliters (mL)

The appropriate formula is:

Weight in Kilograms x Dosage per Kilogram = Dosage required

You first need to convert the 13 pounds to kilogram, and to do this you need to divide that amount by 2.2.

13 pounds ÷ 2.2 = 5.90909 kilograms

Now using the formula you chose:

5.90909 kilograms x 1.5 milligrams per kilogram can be written as:

(5.90909 kilogram x 1.5 milligrams)/1 kilogram

The kilogram units above and below cancel out, and you can now multiply:

5.90909 x 1.5 milligrams, which produces 8.8636 milligrams

For the next stage of calculating the number of milliliters of medication the child should receive, the formula to use is:

Medication ordered / Medication available x Volume per Medication Available = Milliliters Needed

8.8636 milligrams / 75 milligrams x 1 milliliter = Milliliters Needed

The milligram units above and below cancel out completely, and so what remains is:

8.8636 milliliters / 75 whose result is 0.118181 milliliters, and it can be rounded up to 0.12 milliliters (mL)

(23)    The question required that you calculate the amount of medication the nurse was supposed to draw up in order to treat the patient.

The right answer is 4.8mL

You may recognize this question as one of mass versus liquid, and so that is the area from which you need to find the appropriate formula. The relevant formula in this case is:

(Medication ordered / Medication available) x Volume per Medication Available = Milliliters Needed

The calculations will, therefore, look like this:

(20 grams / 25 grams) x 6 milliliters

The gram units above and below will cancel out completely, and when you divide 20 and 25 by the common divisor, 5, you will be left with:

4/5 x 6 milliliters

After you do the multiplication what you will have is 24/5 mL, which works out to 4.8 mL.

(24)   This question required that you find out the quantity of sodium chloride contained in 0.00058 kiloliters of Natural Saline (NS)

The answer is 5.2 grams (g)

In this question, the challenge is to do calculations involving amounts within given IV fluids. For this particular question, the formula you need to apply is:

(Percentage of concentration) / 100 x Volume in milliliters (mL) = Dosage needed in grams(g)

It is important to remember also that Natural Saline (NS) has sodium chloride in concentration level of 0.9%. At the same time, the doctor's medication order is provides the dosage in kiloliters, yet the formula to use works with milliliters. As such, there is need to convert the kiloliters to milliliters.

Converting kiloliters to milliliters requires that you multiply the amount given by the doctor by 1,000 to get the amount in liters, and multiply further by 1,000 to find the accurate amount in milliliters.

0.00058 kiloliters x 1,000 = 0.58 liters, and 0.58 liters x 1,000 = 580 milliliters.

You can now proceed to work with the dosage formula as shown below:

0.9%/100 x 580 milliliters (mL) = (0.9/100 x 100/100) x 580 milliliters

You will have the 100 over 100 canceling out completely, to remain with:

0.9/100 x 580 milliliters

Multiply the above units to get 522 milliliters, and then divide that amount with the 100 that is the denominator to get 5.22 milliliters or simply 5.2 milliliters (mL).

Alternatively, divide 580 by 100 to get 5.80, and then multiply across to get 0.9 x 5.8mL. The answer will still be 5.22mL or 5.2mL.

(25)   This question required that you calculate the rate of flow of the IV ordered by the doctor, given the amount and the period it should take to give it to the patient via an infusion pump.

The right answer is 26.9 milliliters per hour.

This question requires that you understand how to deal with volume versus time and IV rate, and so the appropriate formula to use is:

Volume in milliliters / Time in hours = Rate of Flow in milliliters per hour (mL/hr)

For your calculations to be smooth, you need to work with like-terms. So you need to begin by converting the amount in kiloliters to amount in milliliters. You can do this through a 2-stage multiplication, first changing the kL to L and then the L to mL.

0.00014 kiloliters x 1,000 x 1,000 = 140 milliliters (mL)

The formula you identified can now work as shown below:

140 milliliters / 5.2 hours = Rate of Flow in milliliters per hour (mL/hr)

The answer is 26.923 milliliters per hour or simply 26.9mL/hr.

(26)    This question required that you calculate the number of milliliters the nurse needs to administer to the patient, given the weight of the medication and that of the pediatric patient.

The answer is 0.06 milliliters (mL)

The first step is to establish the dosage the child should be given in weight, and the appropriate formula to use when dealing with dosage provided in weights is:

Weight in Kilograms x Dosage per Kilogram = Needed Dosage

Substituting the figures provided in the medical order:

The infant weighs 3kg

For each kilogram, you should give 2.5mg

So, for 3kg you need to give 2.5mg x 3, which is 7.5mg.

However, the question asks for the amount of liquid in milliliters to be given to the infant. So, you must use a formula that deals with both mass and liquid since you have established the infant requires 7.5mg of medication.

The appropriate formula to use at this stage is:

Amount ordered / Amount available x Volume per Available = Amount of Liquid Required

(7.5 milligrams /125 milligrams) x 1 milliliter = milliliters required

You can begin by canceling out the milligram units, and when you multiply the remaining fraction by 1 milliliter you will have:

7.5/125 milliliters, and this works out to 0.06 milliliters (mL).

(27) This question required that you calculate the number of tablets to be given to the patient, when the medication record has dosage in kilograms.

The right answer for this question is 1 ½ tablets.

Workings

The appropriate formula for solving this problem is:

Amount ordered / Amount available = Number of tablets available

This may look easy, but you need to remember to make the units you are to work with uniform, considering the amount ordered is in kilograms while the amount available is in micrograms.

To convert kilograms to micrograms, you will have to multiply twice by 1,000, the first time to convert kilograms to grams and the second time to convert grams to micrograms. The conversion calculations will go like this:

0.015 kilograms x 1,000 x 1,000 = 15,000 micrograms

Now using the formula you identified:

15,000 mcg / 10,000 mcg = Number of tablets available

The mcg units cancel out completely, and when you divide 15,000 by 10,000 you get one and a half tablets or 1½ tablets.

(28)   This question required that you find out the rate of flow of dopamine infused and provide the answer in milliliters per hour (mL/hr).

The right answer is 274.7 milliliters per hour (mL/hr)

The assumption here is that you can work with mass and time as well as IV rate all in the case of one patient. First you need to identify the most appropriate formula to work with, and where there is need to convert units for uniformity, you use the correct factor. The most convenient formula to use here is:

(Amount ordered per hour / Amount available) x Volume in milliliters = Rate of IV flow in mL/hr

Now convert the micrograms per hour (mcg/hr) to milligrams per hour (mg/hr). To do this you need to divide the value you have by 1,000 as follows:

14,221 micrograms (mcg) ÷ 1,000 = 14.221 milligrams (mg)

So now you are going to work with rate of infusion as 14.221 milligrams per hour.

Back to the formula for calculating IV rate:

$$\frac{14.221 \; milligrams \; per \; Hour}{17.5 \; milligrams} \; \text{x 338 milliliters = Rate of IV flow in mL/hr}$$

For starters, the milligram units can cancel each other out and disappear, and when you multiply the remaining numbers you will have:

(4.806.698 milliliters per hour / 17.5), which works to 274.668 milliliters per hour, and this you can round to 274.7 milliliters per hour (mL/hr).

(29)    The requirement for this question was that you calculate the rate of flow of the IV in terms of gtts/min.

The right answer for this question is 21gtts/min.

The appropriate formula to apply here is:

(Volume in milliliters / Time in minutes) x Drop factor in gtts per mL = Rate of IV flow in gtts/min

After noticing that the period over which to infuse the fluid has been provided in hours yet the formula works with minutes, you must do the necessary conversion as follows:

14.6 hours x 60 = 876 minutes

Back to the formula, your calculations will look like this:

(744 milliliters / 876 minutes) x 25 gtts per milliliter (gtts/mL) = (744 milliliters / 876 minutes) x (25 gtts / 1 milliliter)

You can begin by cancelling out the milliliter units diagonally, and then multiplying the remainder of the two fractions. At this point you will have:

18,600 gtts / 876 = 21.2328gtts per minute, and because you cannot divide drops for the sake of infusion, the answer will be 21gtts/min.

(30)   This question required that you calculate the rate of IV flow in terms of milliliters per hour (mL/hr), in order to maintain the appropriate levels of fluid for a child who weighs 27 kilogram.

The right answer for this question is 68.33 milliliters per hour (mL/hr)

To succeed in answering this question, it is important that you remember the schedule that shows the required level of fluid per given age group. For someone weighing 27kg, the requirement is for the people whose weight range from 20kg to 70kg.

Anyone whose weight falls within this range needs to automatically be allocated 1,500 milliliters of fluid. Then for every kilogram of weight over and above 20 kilograms, the person should get an additional 20 milliliters. So, for this child, the equation that would produce the correct answer looks like this:

Required amount of fluids = 1,500mL + ((27kg – 20kg) x 20mL)

In short, subtract 20kg from 27kg and what you get you multiply by 20mL. You then need to add that output to the basis 1,500mL to get the total amount of fluid to give a 27kg child.

1,500mL + (7 x 20mL) = 1,500mL x 140mL = 1640mL

Now that you have established the exact amount the child requires in milliliters, you need to identify the formula appropriate for calculating the rate of IV flow. This formula is:

Volume in milliliters / Time in hours = Required rate of IV flow in mL/hr

In this question, the formula will work like this:

1,640 milliliters / 24 hours

You will be using 24 hours as the divisor because the amount of fluid you are working with is the recommendation per day, and the day is made up of 24 hours.

1,640 milliliters / 24 hours = 68.3333mL/hr or simply 68.33mL/hr

(31)    This question required that you calculate the rate of IV flow in terms of milliliters per hour for a child whose weight is 16 kilograms.

The right answer for this question is 54.17 milliliters per hour (mL/hr)

<u>Workings</u>

The first step should be to establish the amount of fluid such a child requires each day, and to do that you ought to rely on the standard schedule. Any child whose weight falls within the range, 10kg to 20kg, must automatically have 1,000 milliliters of fluid set aside, and then after that the child should receive 50 milliliters for every kilogram above 10 kilograms. You can build your working formula like this:

1,000mL + ((16 − 10) x 50mL). Once you calculate this you get:

1,000mL + (6 x 50mL), which is 1,000mL + 300mL

The total amount of fluids the child weighing 16kg requires each day is 1,300mL.

On referring back to the question, you will realize the answer required addresses the rate of IV flow per hour. So the suitable formula to use is:

Volume in milliliters / Time in hours x Rate of IV flow in milliliters per hour (mL/hr)

1,300 milliliters / 24 hours = 54.1666 milliliters per hour (mL/hr)

(32)   This question required that you calculate the rate of flow that you need to set for the pump in terms of milliliters per hour, given the medication weight in the fluid and the patient's weight in kilograms.

The right answer for this question is 6.9 milliliters per hour (mL/hr)

The appropriate formula to use here is:

Amount ordered per hour / Amount available x Volume in milliliters = Rate of flow in milliliters per hour

First of all you need to convert order issued per time so that it is in terms of amount needed for this 36kg weighing patient. Remember the patient weighs 36 kilograms and the dosage is given in terms of 10 micrograms per kilogram per hour. In short, the dosage is basically in kilogram terms. To establish the amount of dosage the patient needs, the calculations should be done using the formula:

Patient's weight in kilograms x Dosage per kilogram = Dosage amount needed

36 kilograms @ the rate of 10 micrograms per kilogram per hour = 360 micrograms per hour

The next thing you need to do is convert the 360 micrograms per hour to milligrams per hour, and to do this you are supposed to divide the micrograms by 1,000.

360 micrograms ÷ 1,000 = 0.36 milligrams per hour (mg/hr)

You are now ready to calculate the rate of flow, and to do this you are going to use the formula:

(Amount ordered per hour / Amount available) x Volume in milliliters = Rate of flow in milliliters per hour

(0.36 milligrams per hour / 15.3 milligrams) x 294 milliliters = Rate of flow in milliliters per hour

The milligram units above and below cancel out completely, and as you proceed with the multiplication you will have:

0.36 per hour / 15.3 x 294 milliliters = 6.91764 milliliters per hour

You can round this up as 6.9mL/hr.

(33)   Here you were required to state the amount of fluid in milliliters that a patient weighing 62 pounds needed to take in a day.

The right answer is 1,663.64 milliliters (mL)

Workings

As you search for the appropriate formula, remember this question is assessing your knowledge on fluid maintenance for individuals. As such, you need to recall your schedule of weights so as to see where 62 pounds fit. However, before that you need to convert the pounds to kilograms as the schedule uses kilograms.

62 pounds ÷ 2.2 = 28.181818 kilograms

According to the schedule of weights versus fluids, it is clear this person's weight falls within the range from 20kg to 70kg. Here the person is supposed to automatically receive 1,500mL of fluids, and in addition receive 20 milligrams for every kilogram over and above 20 kilograms.

Considering the person weighs 28.181818kg, your calculations should look like this:

1,500mL + ((28.181818kg – 20kg) @ 20mL), which is:

1,500mL + (8.181818kg @ 20mL), which works to 1,500mL + 163.636363mL

So, in one day, the person weighing 62lb should receive 1,663.636363mL, and you can round that to 1,663.64mL.

(34)    This question required that you calculate the number of tablets the nurse would administer to the patient considering the doctor ordered 12g of Potassium Chloride as in the brand, K-Dur, yet the health institution has stocked the drug in tablets of 12,000mg each.

The right answer for this question is 1 tablet.

The best formula to use in solving this problem of mass versus mass is:

Amount ordered / Amount available = Number of tablets needed

Although you are dealing with mass all through, it is important that the values you are working with be in similar units. For that reason, you could convert the value in milligrams to a value in grams, in which case you divide the value you have by 1,000.

12,000 milligrams ÷1,000 = 12 grams

Amount ordered / Amount available = Number of tablets needed

At this juncture, it is clear that the dosage given by the doctor and the dosage for the available medication is the same; both being 12 grams. You can do the math mentally now, but for calculations' sake:

12 grams / 12 grams has everything cancelling out to leave 1/1 which is 1. So the nurse needed to give the patient just a single tablet.

(35)   This question required that you find out the rate of IV flow for NS measuring 0.26 liters, and which requires infusing over a period of 1,200 minutes, when the drop factor calibration on the infusion set is 3gtts/mL.

The right answer for this question is 1gtts/min.

Clearly this question demands that you have proper understanding of the volume versus time and IV drop rate calculations, including knowledge of the proper formula to use under the circumstances. The appropriate formula is:

Volume in milliliters / Time in minutes x Drop factor in gtts/mL = Required rate of flow in gtts/min

The first thing you need to do is convert the amount ordered from liters to milliliters so as to match the units of the formula. To do this you need to multiply 0.26 liters by 1,000 to turn the value into milliliters.

0.26 liters x 1,000 = 260 milliliters (mL)

Following the formula already identified, the calculations will look like this:

260 milliliters / 1,200 minutes x 3 gtts/mL = Required rate of flow in gtts/min

You can divided by 3 diagonally, so that as 3 results to 1,200 results to 400. Essentially what you will be having at this juncture is:

(260 milliliters / 400 minutes) x 1 gtts / 1 milliliters = Required rate of flow in gtts/min

You can cancel out the milliliter units diagonally, and if you proceed to multiply the fractions across, you will have:

260 gtts / 400 minutes, and this works to 0.65gtts per minute. However, it is not feasible to infuse half a drop at a time, so this decimal value will be rounded upwards to constitute a full drop. Hence the answer is 1gtts/min.

(36) This question required that you calculate the number of milliliters the nurse ought to administer to the child patient of 12kg, considering the doctor's dosage is stated as 2.5mL/kg while the dosage of the hospital medication is in terms of 125mg/2mL.

The right answer is 0.48 milliliters (mL)

Workings

In such a problem involving dosage by weight, the most suitable formula to use is:

Patient's weight in kilograms x Dosage per kilogram = Needed dosage

12 kilograms x 2.5 milligrams per kilogram = Needed dosage

12kg @ 2.5mg per kg = 30mg/kg

Now that you have found the mass dosage, you need to calculate the number of liters that will deliver it in terms of milliliters. The appropriate formula for this is:

(Amount ordered / Amount available) x Volume per Available = Needed Liquid

When you have (30 milligrams / 125 milligrams) x 2 milliliters, you can cancel out the milligram units completely, and then when you divide the numerator and the denominator by 5 as the common divisor, you get:

6/25 x 2 milliliters, and this, after doing the multiplication, gives you 12/25. This, in decimal form, is 0.48 milliliters (mL).

(37)    This question required that you find out the rate of IV flow given the time it takes to infuse 0.0003 kiloliters of 0.9% sodium chloride (NaCl) IV in a period of 10 hours.

The right answer for this question is 40gtts/min.

Workings

For this question dealing with volume versus time as well as the rate of IV drop, the best formula to use is:

(Volume in milliliters / Time in minutes) x Drop factor in gtts per milliliter = rate of flow in gtts per minute

For the calculations to be smooth, it is good that you convert the hours into minutes, so you will be working with the same units the formula has. And since to convert hours to minutes you need to multiply the value you have by 60:

10 hours x 60 = 600 minutes

You will also notice that the doctor has given the dosage in kiloliters yet the formula has milliliters, in which case you need to convert 0.0003 kiloliters to milliliters.

This will involve a two-stage multiplication by 1,000m the first stage producing liters and the next stage producing milliliters. Here is the working:

0.0003 kiloliters x 1,000 = 0.3 liters

0.3 liters x 1,000 = 300 milliliters

Now you are ready to work with the formula:

(Volume in milliliters / Time in minutes) x Drop factor in gtts per milliliter = rate of flow in gtts per minute

(300 milliliters / 600 minutes) x 79gtts per milliliter = rate of flow in gtts per minute

This is the same as:

(300 milliliters / 600 minutes) x (79 gtts x 1 milliliter) = rate of flow in gtts per minute

You can cancel out the milliliter units diagonally and then divided the numerator and denominator by 300. At this point what you will have remained with is:

(½ minutes x 79 gtts / 1) and this works out to 79 gtts / 2 minutes.

After you work out the fraction you get 39.5gtts per minute, and since the answer must be in full drops and the decimal has reached half of ten, you are supposed to give your answer as 40gtts/min.

(38)    In this question you were required to find out the quantity of Sodium Chloride in 0.2 liters NS.

The right answer for this question is 1.8 grams (g)

In this question that is testing how well you understand calculations involving quantities in IV fluids, you need to keep in mind that NS has 0.9% Sodium Chloride, and that the appropriate formula to use is:

(Percentage of Concentration / 100) x Volume in milliliters = Dosage quantity in grams (g)

Begin by converting the 0.2 liters to milliliters because the formula is using milliliters, and you will have:

0.2 liters x 1,000 = 200 milliliters (mL)

Now you can proceed to apply the identified formula and your calculations will look like this:

(0.9% / 100) x 200 milliliters = Dosage quantity in grams (g)

This is the same as (0.9/100 x 100/100) x 200 milliliters

As you do your calculations, 100 over 100 will cancel out completely and so you will now have:

0.9/100 x 200 milliliters = Dosage quantity in grams (g)

Multiply 0.9 x 200 milliliters and you will have 180.0 and when you divide that by the denominator, 100, you will be left with 1.8 milliliters (mL). In short:

(0.9 x 200 milliliters) / 100 = (180 grams / 100) = 1.800 grams or 1.8g.

(39)    This question required that you calculate the rate of IV flow in terms of milliliters per hour (mL/hr)

The right answer for this question is 22.5 milliliters per hour (mL/hr).

Workings

In this question involved with volume versus time and IV rate in milligrams, the best formula to use is:

Volume in milliliters / Time in hours = Rate of IV flow in milliliters per hour (mL/hr)

Begin by converting the time period that is in minutes to time in hours, because the formula uses hours. To change minutes to hours you need to divide the value you have by 60, and so you will have:

1,368 minutes ÷ 60 = 22.8 hours

The next thing you need to do is to convert the dosage provided in microliters to milliliters as the formula in use utilizes milliliters.

514,000 ÷ 1,000 = 514.000 milliliters or 514 milliliters (mL)

Now proceeding with the identified formula:

514 milliliters / 22.8 hours= 22.5 milliliters per hour (mL/hr)

(40)   The question required that you calculate the rate of IV flow in terms of milliliters per hour (mL/hr) given the volume and the period.

The right answer for this question is 77.7 milliliters per hour (mL/hr).

The suitable formula for this kind of problem is:

Volume in milliliters / Time in hours = Rate of IV flow in milliliters per hour (mL/hr)

Since the period over which infusion is to be done has been provided in minutes and the formula to use is in hours, it is important that you convert the minutes to hours by dividing the value given by 60. So you will have:

288 minutes ÷ 60 = 4.8 hours

Now applying the formula you identified as suitable:

373 milliliters / 4.8 hours = Rate of IV flow in milliliters per hour (mL/hr)

Rate of IV flow in milliliters per hour (mL/hr) = 77.708 milliliters per hour, which you can write simply as 77.7 milliliters per hour (mL/hr).

(41)    The question required that you calculate the amount of fluid the nurse needs to give a child in one day if that child weighs 35 kilograms.

The right answer for this question is 1,800 milliliters (mL).

This question seeks to test your understanding of fluid maintenance for different individuals, and for you to tackle it properly you need to remember the schedule that is followed in calculating the amount of liquid for individuals of different body weights.

A child weighing 35 kilograms falls under the category of people weighing from 20 kilograms to 70 kilograms, where such an individual straightaway qualifies for 1,500 milliliters of fluids. Then in addition, you need to add to the person's fluid intake 20 milliliters for every kilogram the person weighs over and above 20 kilograms.

With this information, you can design a suitable formula like this:

Needed fluids in mL = 1,500mL +((35kg – 20kg) @ 20mL).

Needed fluids in mL = 1,500mL + (15kg @ 20mL) = 1,500mL + 300mL

Needed fluids in mL = 1800mL per day

(42)   The question required that you calculate the amount of medication to administer in milliliters.

The right answer for this question is 0.06 milliliters (mL).

Workings

In this dosage per weight question, the appropriate formula to start with is:

Patient's weight in kilograms x Dosage per kilogram = Dosage required

1 kilogram x 2.5 milligrams per kilogram works out as shown below:

1 kilogram x (2.5 milligrams / 1 kilogram), and when the kilogram units cancel each other out diagonally, you are left with 2.5 milligrams. So the dosage required for the infant is 2.5 milligrams (mg).

However, the question requires that you determine the amount of available medication to be dispensed in terms of milliliters. The appropriate formula to apply in this case is:

(Amount ordered / Amount available) x Volume per available = Amount of liquid needed

When you put in the equivalent values, what you have is:

(2.5 milligrams / 125 milligrams) x 3 milliliters = Amount of liquid needed

For starters the milligram units will cancel out completely, and when you divide 2.5 and 125 with 2.5 as the common divisor you will remain with:

1/50 x 3 milliliters = Amount of liquid needed

Once you solve the multiplication you get:

3/50 milliliters or 0.06 milliliters (mL)

(43)   The question required that you find out the quantity of Sodium Chloride contained in 0.00056 kiloliters ¼ NS.

The right answer for this question is 1.3 grams (g).

Workings

In a question like this one dealing with the IV fluid, it is important to remember that the concentration of Sodium Chloride (NaCl) in the Natural Saline solution is 0.9%. Your calculations will therefore proceed as follows:

0.9% x ¼ = 0.225%

In order to establish the right quantity of Sodium Chloride in the solution, you need to use the formula:

(Percentage of Concentration / 100) x Volume in milliliters = Amount in grams

However, since the medication record has volume in kiloliters and the formula uses milliliters, you need to first of all convert the kiloliters to milliliters. This requires that you multiply the value provided by 1,000 twice, first to get the value in liters and the second time to get the value in milliliters.

0.00056 kiloliters x 1,000 = 0.56 liters

0.56 liters x 1,000 = 560 milliliters

Now applying the identified formula:

(0.225%/100) x 560 milliliters = Amount in grams. This is the same as:

(0.225/100 x 100/100) x 560 milliliters = Amount in grams

It is easy to see that 100 over 100 can cancel out completely. Then you can do the necessary multiplications as shown here below:

(0.225 x 560 milliliters) / 100 = 126/100 grams, which works out to 1.26 grams (g)

You can round up the answer to 1.3g.

(44)  The question required that you calculate the rate of IV flow in milliliters per hour when 379 milliliters NS IV has been prescribed to be infused over a period of 1,374 minutes via an infusion pump.

The right answer for this question is 16.6 milliliters per hour (mL/hr).

Workings

For a question like this one dealing with volume versus time as well as IV rate, the appropriate formula is:

First of all you need to convert the minutes representing the period over which infusion will take place to hours.

1,374 minutes ÷ 60 = 22.9 hours

Now back to the identified formula:

(379 milliliters / 22.9 hours) = 16.55 milliliters per hour, which you can round upwards to 16.6 milliliters per hour (mL/hr)

(45)   This question required that you calculate the rate of IV flow in terms of milliliters per hour, given that the doctor's prescription was 0.76liters D5W IV to be infused over a period of 264 minutes.

The right answer for this question is 172.7 milliliters per hour (mL/hr).

Workings

This question, being one of volume versus time and rate of IV flow, you need to use the formula:

The first step should be to convert the units of time from minutes to hours so as to be able to use the values in the identified formula.

264 minutes ÷ 60 = 4.4 hours

The next thing should be to convert the dosage of 0.76 liters to milliliters, which requires that you multiply that value by 1,000.

0.76 liters x 1,000 = 760 milliliters

Now back to the identified formula:

760 milliliters / 4.4 hours = 172.7272 milliliters per hour, and this can be rounded to 172.7 milliliters per hour (mL/hr)

(46)    This question required that you calculate the milliliters of fluid appropriate for a child weighing 56 pounds.

The right answer for this question is 1,609.09 milliliters (mL)

This is a question about fluid maintenance for individuals with varying weights, and the calculations are usually in kilograms and milliliters. As such, any weight given in pounds must be converted to kilograms

56 pound ÷2.2 = 25.4545 kilograms

For a person weighing slightly more than 25kg, the range within which their weight falls is from 20kg to 70kg, and here an individual qualifies for 1,500mL of fluid before any other calculations can be made. It is after that you need to calculate the amount of fluid to be added, considering 20mL is supposed to be administered for every single hour above the first 20kg. You can, therefore, design your equation as shown here below:

Required fluids in mL = 1,500mL + ((25.4545kg − 20kg) @ 20mL)

Required fluids in mL = 1,500mL + (5.4545kg @ 20mL)

Required fluids in mL = 1,500mL + 109.09mL, and this adds up to 1,609.09mL

(47)    The question required that you calculate the rate of IV flow and give the answer in gtts per minute (gtts/min).

The right answer for this question is 21 gtts per minute (gtts/min)

This question that entails calculation of volume versus time and even the rate of IV drop needs to use the formula:

(Volume in milliliters / Time in minutes) x Drop factor in gtts per milliliter – Rate of IV flow in gtts per minute

Using the value in the dosage:

(142 milliliters / 666 minutes) x 97 gtts per milliliter = Rate of IV flow in gtts per minute

You can write this equation as:

(142 milliliters / 666 minutes) x (97 gtts per milliliter / 1 milliliter)= Rate of IV flow in gtts per minute

Outright, the milliliter units cancel out and you are left with:

 (142 x 97 gtts) / 666 minutes, which is (13,774 gtts / 666 minutes) and this can be simplified to 20.68 gtts per minute.

However, drops, represented by gtts, can only be presented in whole units, so the right answer is 21gtts/min.

(48)   This question required that you calculate the number of milliliters of Solumedrol the nurse needs to administer to a patient weighing 25 pounds, when the dosage of the Solumedrol available has been provided as 75 milligrams per milliliter.

The right answer for this question is 0.23 milliliters (mL)

Workings

In this question that deals with dosage in terms of amount per weight, the appropriate formula to apply in establishing the right dosage for the child is:

Weight in Kilograms x Dosage per kilogram = needed dosage

But first you need to ensure the dosage units match those used in the formula, so you need to convert 25 pounds to kilograms. This entails dividing the child's weight in pounds by 2.2.

25 pounds ÷ 2.2 = 11.3636 kilograms

Back to the formula, your equation should look like this:

11.3636 kilogram x 1.5 milligrams per kilogram = needed dosage

(11.3636 kilogram x 1.5 milligram) / kilogram = needed dosage

Cancel out the kilogram units beneath and above, and then multiply the remaining figures. What you get is:

11.3636 x 1.5 milligrams = 17.04545 milligrams (mg)

The next step is to calculate the amount of liquid Solumedro to be administered based on the dosage amount you have just calculated. This calculation should be based on the formula:

(Amount ordered / Amount available) x Volume per available = needed liquid

(17.04545 milligrams / 75 milligrams) x 1 milliliter = needed liquid

The milligram units will automatically cancel each other out, and when you do the rest of the multiplication you will get:

(17.04545 milligrams / 75)= 0.227272 milliliters or simply 0.23mL.

(49)   This question required that you calculate the number of tablets to administer to the patient given the medication record reads Potassium Chloride, as in the drug, K-Dur, and the dosage is 0.022 kilograms.

The right answer for this question is one tablet.

This being a question dealing with mass to mass calculations, the appropriate formula is:

Amount ordered / Amount available = Number of tablets needed

First convert the 23 grams to kilograms, and to do this you need to divide by 1,000.

23 grams ÷ 1,000 = 0.023 kilograms (kg)

Now, following the identified formula of , Amount ordered / Amount available

0.022 kilograms / 0.023 kilograms = 0.988. You can round this upwards so that the answer is one tablet.

(50)    In this question you were required to convert 40° Celsius to Fahrenheit.

The answer is C. 104°F

Workings

When you want to convert degrees Celsius to degrees Fahrenheit the formula is:

(0°C × 9/5) + 32°

In this case, the degrees to be converted are 40°C, so:

(40° x 9/5)+32°

Divide diagonally and you will get rid of the denominator, 5, then instead of 40° you will have 8°. Now you have:

(8° x 9) + 32°, which becomes 72° + 32° and the answer is 104°F.

(51) In this question you were required to convert 15°C to degrees Fahrenheit.

The correct answer is A. 59°F.

<u>Workings</u>

Using the formula:

(0°C × 9/5) + 32°, substitute for 0°C and you will have:

(15° x 9/5) + 32°

You can divide by 5 diagonally, so that you have 3° in place of 15° and 1 in place of the denominator, 5. What you have now looks like this:

(3° x 9) + 32° = (27° + 32°)F, which adds up to 59°F.

(52)   In this question you were required to convert 52°C to Fahrenheit.

The answer for this question is D. 126°F

<u>Workings</u>

Using the formula:

(0°C × 9/5) + 32°, you will have (52° x 9/5) + 32° after fillin in the degrees Celsius.

The rest of the working will look like this:

(52° x 9)/5 + 32°, which works to 93.6° +32°

So the answer is 125.6°F, which can be rounded up to 126°F.

(53)    In this question, you were required to convert 23.5° Celsius to Fahrenheit.

The correct answer for this question is B. 74°F.

Workings

Using the formula, (0°C × 9/5) + 32°, you will have:

(23.5°C × 9/5) + 32°, which is (23.5° x 9)/5 + 32°

Further calculations will give you 211.5°/5 + 32°

This works out to 42.3° + 32°, which totals 74.3° Fahrenheit. You can round this downwards to have your answer as 74°.

(54) This question required that you convert 32° Celsius to Fahrenheit.

The correct answer for this question is A. 90°F.

<u>Workings</u>

Using the formula, (0°C × 9/5) + 32°, you will have:

(32°C × 9/5) + 32°, which is (32° x 9)/5+ 32°

(32° x 9)/5+ 32° = (288°/5)+ 32°, which works out to 57.6° + 32°.

The answer is, therefore, 89.6° Fahrenheit, and which you can round upwards to 90°F.

(55)   This question required that you convert 100° Fahrenheit to Celsius.

The correct answer for this question is C. 38° Celsius.

<u>Workings</u>

Whenever you want to convert degrees Fahrenheit to degrees Celsius, the formula to use is:

°C = (°F – 32°) x 5/9

In this question, therefore, your working will look like this:

(100° – 32°) x 5/9

This gives you 68° x 5/9which you can express as (68° x 5) / 9

After multiplying the figures above, you will have 340°/9 that after simplification becomes 37.777° Celsius. You can round this figure upwards so that your answer becomes 38° Celsius.

(56)   This question required that you convert 55° Fahrenheit to degrees Celsius.

The correct answer for this question is D. 13° Celsius.

Workings

Following the formula:

°C = (°F − 32°) x 5/9

$(55° − 32°) \times 5/9 = 23° \times \frac{5}{9}$, which works out to 12.777° Celsius

You can round up this number to 13° Celsius.

(57)   This question required that you convert 60° Fahrenheit to degrees Celsius.

The correct answer for this question is C. 16°C

Workings

Using the formula, °C = (°F − 32°) x 5/9:

(60° − 32°) x 5/9 = 28° x 5/9, which works to (28° x 5) / 9

This further works to 140°/9, which, when you calculate gives 15.555° Celsius.

You can round up this answer to 16° Celsius.

(58) This question required that you convert 39° Fahrenheit to degrees Celsius.

The correct answer for this question is B. 4°C

Using the formula, °C = (°F − 32°) x 5/9:

°C = (39° − 32°) x 5/9, which works to 7° x 5/9

After you do the necessary multiplication, your fraction becomes 35°/9.

35° divided by 9 produces 3.8888°F, and you can round this to 4°F.

(59)  This question required that you convert 78° Fahrenheit to degrees Celsius.

The correct answer for this question is A. 26°C

Using the formula, °C = (°F – 32°) x 5/9:

°C = (78° – 32°) x 5/9, which works to 46° x 5/9

After doing the necessary multiplication, the fraction you get is 230/9, and the subsequent division produces 25.555 or 26°C.

(60)   You were expected to state the Arabic number that is written as LXXVII using Roman numerals.

Answer Choices:

A.  57

B.  77

C.  27

D.  527

The correct answer for this question is B. 77.

Explanation

In this question you look at the Roman numerals with the greatest value and find it is L that represents 50, and then you add the value immediately next to it to the right, which is XX representing 20. Your value then becomes 50+20, which is 70. But then before you are done you notice that next to XX there is VII, which represents (5+2) or simply 7, and so you add it to the other value you had. So now you have 50+20+7, which totals 77.

(61) The question required that you state the amount represented by the numeral written in Roman as IVss?

Answer Choices:

A. 6 1/2

B. 4

C. 4 ½

D. 15

The correct answer is C. 4 ½

Explanation

In this question you look at the Roman number provided and notice the numeral with the greatest value is V, which represents 5. To the left of V is I that represents 1. The rules guiding the writing of Roman numbers indicate that any numeral to the left of a bigger value than itself is to be subtracted from that bigger value, and for that reason you need to subtract one from five. You now have the value as 4, but you still have 'ss' immediately after it. 'ss' stands for 'half' in the medical jargon, and so the full value as required by the question is 4½

(62)    The question required that you state the number of times in a day, or essentially a 24hr period, a nurse should administer medication to a patient if the patient's medication order reads 'gtt II o.s. tid'.

Answer Choices:

A.  Three

B.  Eleven

C.  Once

D.  Two

The correct answer is A. Three.

<u>Explanation</u>

In the language used in the medical field, 't.i.d.' in indication of three times a day.

(63)    This question required that you calculate the value of X as used in the equation, 3X = 51.

Answer Choices:

A.  51

B.  3

C.  17

D.  4

The correct answer is C. 17

<u>Working</u>

When you have been given 3x = 51 and your ultimate goal is to find the value represented by x, you work towards segregating x, which is the unknown value, so that it remains on one side of the equation alone.

In this particular case, in order to leave X alone as opposed to having it remain as 3x, you divide that side by 3, so that you now have 3x/3.

But then, in such questions what you do the left side of the equation you must also do to the right. So you need to divide the right side by 3 as well, in which case you will have 51/3. Essentially, this is what you will have at this juncture:

3x/3 = 51/3

3x divided by 3 gives you x, while 51 divide by 3 gives you 17. In short:

x = 17

(64)   In this question, you were required to calculate the value of X in the equation, 1/2 X = 5mg

Answer Choices:

A.  1mg

B.  10mg

C.  0.5mg

D.  5.5mg

The correct answer is B. 10mg.

<u>Working</u>

Given ½ x = 5mg, you need to follow the same principle as in the previous problem, where you worked towards leaving the 'unknown' on its side alone. In this case, if you want remove ½ from ½ x, you ought to divide that number by ½.

You also need to remember that what you do to the left side you need to also do to the right, and vice-versa. So you need to divide the right side by a half as well. You will now have:

½ ÷ ½x= 5mg ÷ ½. This basically means:

½ x 2/1x = 5mg x 2/1

There is a basic rule in math that stipulates that if you are trying to divide a number by a fraction, you can always substitute the division with multiplication on condition you invert the fraction. This is what has happened in these calculations.

The numbers on the left side now cancel out, one by one and two by two, and that is how you are left with x on its own. As for the right side, you can only multiply 5mg by 2, as the answer does not change by dividing the value you get by 1. You will now have 10mg on the right and your equation will look like this:

x = 10mg

(65)   Calculate the value of X in the equation, 0.5x + 1 = 2

Answer Choices:

A.  0.10

B.  1.5

C.  ½

D.  2

The correct answer for this question is D. 2

<u>Working</u>

For the equation, 0.5x + 1 = 2, you need to first of all get rid of the constant on the left, which is 1, and because it is a plus you can only get rid of it by introducing a plus of the same value on that side. For balancing purposes, you also need to introduce a minus 1 on the right side. Effectively you will have:

0.5x +1 − 1 = 2 -1

On the left side the ones cancel out completely while on the right side you remain with 1; meaning 0.5x =1.

You can now proceed to solve for x as you did in the previous questions as follows:

0.5x/0.5 = 1/0.5

One thing you need to know is that 0.5x means 0.5 times x or 0.5 X x. So, the 0.5 above and below cancel out completely, leaving x alone while on the right side you have 1 ÷ 0.5. Keep in mind that 0.5 is the same as a half. So you can write 1 ÷ 0.5 as:

1 ÷ 1/2 which is the same as 1 x 2/1, which works out to 2. Your equation is now x = 2 and that is the answer.

(66)  This question required that you calculate the value of x in the equation, 2.5mg = 1/4x

Answer Choices:

A.  2.5

B.  10mg

C.  10

D.  10mcg

The correct answer for this question is B. 10mg.

<u>Workings</u>

2.5mg = 1/4x

One thing worth noting is it does not matter which side the unknown is, you need to work towards segregating it; leaving it on its own. In this case since the right has a quarter times x, you can introduce 'divide by a quarter' on the same side and then do the same to the left. Your equation will now look like this:

2.5mg ÷ 1/4 = 1/4 ÷ ¼x , and this is the same as 2.5mg x 4/1 = 4/1 x 1/4x After the multiplications, you will now have the equation:

10mg = x. This is the same as x = 10mg.

(67)    The question required that you calculate the appropriate amount in milliliters of Promethazine Hydrochloride injection to be administered to a patient if the dosage on the label is 25mg/ml and the patient requires 12.5mg of the drug.

Answer Choices:

A.  0.5mL

B.  25mL

C.  37.5mL

D.  6.25mL

The correct answer for this question is A. 5mL.

Workings

If 1mL contains 25mg, how many mL will contain 12.5mg?

1ml/25mg x 12.5mg

If you begin by dividing diagonally, 12.5mg divided by itself gives you 1 and when you use it as the divisor for 25mg you get 2. So your new fraction is now:

1ml/2 or ½ mL, which is the same as 0.5mL

(68)   The question required that you calculate the number of grams contained in the drug, Thiabendazole, which fills a bottle whose volume is 120mL and whose label indicates 500mg/5cc.

Answer Choices:

A.  100g

B.  0.01g

C.  12g

D.  12,000g

The correct answer for this question is C. 12g.

Workings

It is important to note that 1c.c. is equal to 1mL, with the variation being that when dealing with solids you use c.c. while when dealing with fluids you use mL. Of course, while mL stands for milliliters c.c. stands for cubic centimeters.

If in 5cc there are 500mg, how many mg are there in 120mL? The equivalent of 120mL is 120c.c. Now calculate the number of mg in one c.c. It is:

500mg/5cc= 100mg/c.c.

If one c.c. has 100mg, how many mg are there in 120c.c.? It is:

100mg x 120 = 12,000mg

However, the question asks for the answer in grams, and so you need to convert 12,000mg to grams by dividing by 1,000.

12,000 ÷ 1,000 = 12g

(69)  The question required that you calculate the number of milligrams that make up 0.5 grams.

Answer Choices:

A. 500mg.

B. 5mg.

C. 5,000mg.

D. 0.0005mg.

The correct answer for this question is A. 500mg.

Workings:

1g = 1,000mg

Therefore, 0.5g = 0.5g x 1,000, which is 500mg.

(70) This question required that you calculate the number of liters comprising 27.3 milliliters.

Answer Choices:

A. 2,730 liters.

B. 0.273 liters.

C. 0.0273 liters.

D. 27,300 liters.

The answer is B. 0.0273 liters.

Workings:

One liter is made up of 1,000 milliliters. This means:

1mL = 1/1,000L

Therefore, 27.3mL = 1/1,000 L x 27.3 = 0.0273L

(71) Find out the number of milliliters comprising eight fluid ounces.

Answer Choices:

A. 240mL

B. 128mL

C. 120mL

D. 3.75mL

The correct answer is A. 240mL.

Workings:

In general, one US fluid ounce comprises 29.574 milliliters. So, if:

1 fluid ounce = 29.574 milliliters, it means:

8 fluid ounces = 29.574 milliliters x 8, which works out to 236.592 milliliters. After rounding the figure upwards to the nearest ten, the answer is 240mL.

(72)    This question required that you calculate the number of milliliters in 3 pints.

Answer Choices

A. 1,950 mL

B. 90mL

C. 1,419 mL

D. 195 mL

The correct answer for this question is C. 1,419mL.

Workings:

There are generally 473.176 milliliters in one US pint. Therefore, if:

1 US pint = 473.176mL

3 US pints = 473.176mL x 3 = 1,419.528mL

This answer, rounded downwards, is 1,419mL.

(73)  The hospital pharmacy has the injection drug, Chlordiazepoxide hydrochloride, as in the brand, Librium, which is supplied in dry powder form. The medication comes in packets of 100mg, accompanied by a separate vial of 2mL diluent. You are required to find out the number of such vials that should be opened in order to dilute a dose of 30mg of the drug.

Answer Choices:

A.  3

B.  1

C.  10

D.  2

The correct answer for this question is B. 1.

Workings:

100mg matches 2mL or 1 vial

How many mL and how many vials would 1mg match? It will be:

2ml/100mg

Then, how many milliliters and how many vials would be needed for 30mg?

2ml/100mg x 30mg

Calculating diagonally, the mg units cancel out completely, so that you are left with:

2ml/100mg x 30, and it works out to 60ml/100 or 0.6mL

Since the diluents comes in 2mL vials and 0.6mL is less than 2mL, only one vial will be opened for the sake of diluting 30mg of the given drug.

(74)    How many mL are there in 9oz?

Answer choices:

0.3mL

2.7mL

270mL

0.27mL

The correct answer for this question is C.270mL

Workings:

1oz = 30mL

Therefore, the number of mL in 9oz is:

30mL x 9 = 270mL

(75)    How many mcg are there in 27mg?

Answer Choices:

370mcg

2,700mcg

27,000mcg

0.0027mcg

The correct answer for this question is C. 27,000mcg.

Workings:

1mg = 1,000mcg

Therefore, 27mg = 1,000mcg x 27 = 27,000mcg.

(76)   How many ounces are there in 15 milliliters?

Answer Choices:

15 ounces

½ ounce

30 ounces

2 ounces

The correct answer for this question is B. ½

Workings:

1oz = 30mL or 30mL = 1oz

Therefore, to find out the ounces comprising 15 milliliters:

1 oz / 30ml x 15mL

Divide diagonally by 15mL, and so 15mL becomes 1 and the denominator, 30mL becomes 2. The ultimate result is 1 oz /2, which is the same as ½ oz or 0.50z.

(77)    How many mg are there in 956mcg?

Answer Choices:

96mg

9,560mg

0.0096mg

0.96mg

The correct answer for this question is D. 0.96mg.

Workings:

1,000 mcg = 1 mg

1 mcg = 1mg / 1,000 mcg

Therefore, 956 mcg = (1mg / 1,000 mcg) x 956 mcg

You can straightaway cancel out the mcg units diagonally, and after multiplying across you will have:

956mg/1,000, and this is the same as 0.956 mg. Once you round the results upwards you get 0.96 mg.

(78)　Calculate the number of ounces in 29½ milliliters of liquid.

Answer Choices:

29.5 oun

885 ounces

0.98 ounces

30 ounces

The correct answer for this question is C. 0.98 ounces.

Workings:

1 oz = 30mL

30 milliliters = 1 ounces

Therefore 1 milliliter = 1 ounce / 30 milliliters

29½ milliliters = 1 ounce / 30 milliliters x 29½ milliliters

You can straightaway cancel out the milliliter units, and what will remain is:

(1 ounce x 29.5) / 30

This works to 29.5 ounces / 30, which works out to 0.983 ounces. This can be rounded down to 0.98 ounces.

(79)    How many mL are there in 10 cc?

Answer Choices:

2.5 milliliters

10 milliliters

0.5 milliliters

None of the choices provided

The correct answer for this question is B. 10 milliliters.

Workings:

ImL or milliliter = 1 cc or 1 cubic centimeter

Therefore 10cc = 10mL or milliliters.

(80)   Calculate the number of milliliters in 5.25 ounces.

Answer Choices:

6 milliliters

3.5 milliliters

157.5 milliliters

5 milliliters

The correct answer for this question is C. 157.5 milliliters.

Workings:

1 oz = 30mL

Therefore 5.25oz = 30mL x 5.25; and this works out to 157.5 milliliters.

(81)   How many cc are there in 35mL?

Answer Choices:

350 cc

3,500 cc

17.5 cc

35 cc

The correct answer to this question is D. 35 cc.

Workings

1 mL = 1 cc

Therefore 35mL is equivalent to 35 x 1 = 35 cc.

(82)  How many milliliters (mL) are there in 7 teaspoons (tsp)?

Answer Choices:

35 milliliters

7 milliliters

0.7 milliliters

5 milliliters

The correct answer for this question is A. 35 milliliters.

The first thing to consider is that 1 teaspoon = 5 milliliters

Therefore, 7 teaspoons = 5 milliliters x 7, and this works out to 35 milliliters (mL).

(83)    How man milliliters are there in 5 liters?

Answer Choices:

5 milliliters

5,000 milliliters

0.005 milliliters

50 milliliters

The correct answer for this question is B. 5,000 milliliters.

Workings

1 liter = 1,000 milliliters

As such, 5 liters = 5 x 1,000 milliliters; and that works out to 5,000 milliliters.

(84)   How many teaspoons are made up of 55 milliliters?

Answer Choices:

275 teaspoons

11 teaspoons

5.5 teaspoons

0.55 teaspoons

The correct answer for this question is B. 11 teaspoons.

Workings

5 milliliters = 1 teaspoon

Therefore, 1 milliliter = 1/ 5 milliliters

It follows that the number of teaspoons in 55 milliliters is:

1/5 milliliters x 55 milliliters

Begin by calculating diagonally, and the denominator will disappear while 55ml will become plain 11. Multiply 11 by 1 across and the answer still remains 11. These are 11 teaspoons.

(85)  How many liters comprise 19 milliliters?

Answer Choices:

0.019 liters

19,000 liters

190 liters

1.9 liters

The correct answer for this question is A. 0.019 liters.

Remember 1,000 milliliters = 1 liter

This means 1 milliliter = 1/1,000 liter

Therefore, 19 milliliters =1/1,000 liter x 19, which is (1 liter x 19) / 1,000

This works out to 19/1,000 or 0.019 liters.

(86)   Calculate the number of milligrams that comprise 4½ grams.

Answer Choices:

4,500 milligrams

4.5 milligrams

0.045 milligrams

7 milligrams

The correct answer for this question is A. 4,500 milligrams.

Workings:

1 gram (g) = 1,000 milligrams (mL)

Therefore, 4 1/2 grams = 1,000 milliliters x 4 1/2  or 1,000 milliliters x 4.5

This works out to 4,500 milligrams.

(87) How many grams are made up of 1,200 micrograms?

Answer Choices:

1.2 grams

1,200 grams

0.0012 grams

12 grams

The correct answer for this question is C. 0.0012 grams.

Workings

The first thing to remember is:

1 gram = (1,000 x 1,000) micrograms

The reason is that by multiplying by the first 1,000 you convert the grams into milligrams, and only when you multiply a second time by 1,000 do you get the number of micrograms in the grams.

This means 1 microgram = 1/1,000,000 grams

Hence, 1,200 micrograms = 1/1,000,000 grams

x 1,200

This works out to 1,200 /1,000,000 grams, which is essentially, 0.001200 grams or 0.0012g.

(88)   How many mcg make 9g?

Answer Choices:

90 mcg

9,000 mcg

0.009 mcg

9,000,000 mcg

The correct answer for this question is D. 9,000,000 mcg.

<u>Workings</u>

1 gram (g) = (1 x 1,000) milligrams (mg), which is 1,000 milligrams

1,000 milligrams x 1,000 = 1,000,000 micrograms (mcg)

This means 1 gram (g) = 1,000,000 micrograms (mcg)

Therefore, 9 grams = 1,000,000 micrograms x 9, and this makes 9,000,000 mcg.

(89)    How many grams comprise 68 micrograms?

Answer Choices:

0.000068 grams

68,000 grams

0.0068 grams

14 grams

The correct answer for this question is A. 0.000068 grams.

The formula to base your calculations on is:

1 microgram = 1/1,000,000 gram

Therefore, 68 micrograms = 1/1,000,000 gram x 68

This works out to (1 x 68) / 1,000,000 grams, which is 68/1,000,000 grams or 0.000068 grams (g).

(90) How many milliliters are in 6 teaspoons?

Answer Choices:

30 milliliters

1/6 milliliters

0.6 milliliters

5 milliliters

The correct answer for this question is A. 30 milliliters.

<u>Workings</u>

1 teaspoon = 5 milliliters

Therefore 6 teaspoons = 5 milliliters x 6, and this works out to 30 milliliters.

(91)    How many liters are there in 9 teaspoons?

Answer Choices:

0.009 liters

45 liters

0.045 liters

450 liters

The correct answer for this question is C. 0.045 liters.

Workings

First of all consider that 1 teaspoon = 5 milliliters

It also means that 1 teaspoon = (5 ÷ 1,000) liters = 0.005 liters

Therefore, 9 teaspoons = 0.005 liters x 9, and this works out to 0.045 liters.

(92)   Calculate the number of cc in 12L.

Answer Choices:

0.012 L

12,000 cc

5,000 cc

12 cc

The correct answer to this question is B. 12,000 cc.

Workings

It is important to remember that 1 cc = 1 mL

And since 1 L = ( 1 x 1,000 ) mL, it follows that 1 L is also ( 1 x 1,000 ) cc.

As such, 12 L = ( 1 x 1,000 ) x 12; and this works to 12,000 cc.

(93)    How many ounces (oz) are there in 16 milliliters (mL)?

Answer Choices:

16000 ounces

0.54 ounces

0.16 ounces

530 ounces

The correct answer for this question is B. 0.54 ounces.

<u>Workings</u>

If you can recall, 1 ounce is made up of 29.574 milliliters. So, if:

29.574 milliliters = 1 ounce

1 milliliter = 1/29.574 ounces

Therefore, 16 milliliters = (1/29.574) x 16 ounces.

This works out to 0.541 ounces or simply 0.54 ounces.

(94)    Calculate the number of kilograms comprising 250 pounds.

Answer Choices:

113.6 kilograms

550 kilograms

0.025 kilograms

2.5 kilograms

The correct answer is A. 113.6 kilograms.

Workings

1 kilogram = 2.2 pounds

1 pound = 1 / 2.2 kilograms

Therefore, 250 pounds = 1 / 2.2 kilograms x 250

This works out to 113.6363 kilograms, and you can round this up to 113.64 kilograms.

(95)    Calculate the number of pounds contained in 195 kilograms.

Answer Choices:

429 pounds

195,000 pounds

0.0195 pounds

88.64 pounds

The correct answer for this question is 429 pounds.

Workings

1 kilogram = 2.2 pounds

Therefore, 195 kilograms = 195 kilograms x 2.2

This works out to 429 pounds.

(96)    Calculate the number of milligrams comprising 9 micrograms.

Answer Choices:

0.009 milligrams

9,000 milligrams

0.001 milligrams

9 milligrams

The correct answer for this question is A. 0.009 milligrams.

Workings

1 milligram = 1,000 micrograms

1 microgram = 1/1,000 milligram

Therefore, 9 micrograms = 1/1,000 micrograms x 9

This works to (1 x 9)/1,000 milligrams, and this becomes 9/1,000 milligrams, which is the same as 0.009 milligrams.

(97)   Calculate the number of milliliters contained in 26 ounces.

Answer Choices:

26,000 milliliters

769 milliliters

0.769 milliliters

13 milliliters

The correct answer for this question is B. 769 milliliters.

Workings

1 ounce = 29.574 milliliters

Therefore, 26 ounces = 29.574 milliliters x 26, and this works to 768.924 milliliters.

You can round this upwards to become 769 milliliters.

(98)   Find out the number of liters that comprise 360 milliliters.

Answer Choices:

36,000 liters

720 liters

0.36 liters

0.0027 liters

The correct answer for this question is C. 0.36 liters.

Workings

1 Liter = 1,000 milliliters

1 milliliter = 1/1,000 Liters

Therefore, 360 milliliters = 1/1,000Liters x 360, and this works out to 360/1,000 Liters

You can also write this fraction as 0.36 liters.

(99) In this question you are required to find out how much Amoxicillin a nurse needs to draw up in order to have 23000 mg of Amoxicillin, bearing in mind that Amoxicillin is available as 1,000,000 mcg per 9ml.

We require the Amoxicillin in mg.

1,000mcg = 1mg

If

1,000mcg        = 1mg

1,000,000 mcg   =?

We cross multiply to get how many mgs are in 1,000,000 mcg.

(1,000,000mcg / 1,000mcg) x 1mg = 1,000mg

The above workings can be interpreted to mean that Amoxicillin can also be found as 1,000 mg per 9ml.

Since we have converted the values to similar units, we can proceed and find how much the nurse requires drawing up in order to get 23,000 mg of Amoxicillin.

1,000 mg      = 9ml

23,000 mg       = ?

We cross multiply to get the amount of liquid required in ml as shown below:

(23,000 mg/1,000) x 9ml = 207ml

The correct answer for this question is therefore 207 ml.

(100)  This question requires you to calculate the flow rate in mL/hr, where a patient is to be given 18.8 mg of dopamine which is available in 363 mL of D5W which is to be infused at the rate of 13,175 mcg/hr.

We start by converting the rate from mcg/hr to mg/hr. This is done by converting mcg to mg.

1,000 mcg = 1mg

Mcg = mg (divide by 1,000)

If

1,000 mcg = 1mg

We cross-multiply as follows:

13,175 mcg / 1,000 mcg x 1mg = 13.175 mg

The working now becomes easier and more accurate because we have converted the values to similar units, i.e. mg. It is important to note that the rate can now be stated as 13.175mg/hr.

Hence

18.8 mg represents 363 Ml

If we cross-multiply the above we have:

 (13.175 milligrams/hour/18.8milligrams) x 363 milliliters = 254.389 ml/hr

The correct answer in this question is therefore 254.389 ml/hr.

(101)   In this question we are required to find out how many mL of Solumedrol a nurse should administer to a child who weighs 29 kg, if Solumedrol is available as 125mg/ 3 ml and it was ordered as 2.5 mg/kg.

We start by calculating the amount of Solumedrol required for 29 kgs. This is done by multiplying 2.5 mg/kg by 29kgs as shown below:

1 kg represents 2.5 mg/kg

Therefore, we cross-multiply

(2.5 milligram/kilogram)/1 kilogram x 29 kilogram = 72.5 milligrams

It is now clear that we want to get the amount of Solumedrol in mL that will give us 72.5 mg, bearing in mind that Solumedol is available as 125mg/ 3 mL.

If,

125mg represents 3 mL

72.5mg = ?

We cross-multiply as follows,

 (72.5mg / 125mg) x 3 ml = 1.74ml

The correct answer for this question is 1.74 mL.

(102) In this question you are required to calculate the number of tablets a nurse should administer in order to achieve 9,000,000 mcg of Ampicillin, if Ampicillin is available as 20g tablets.

We can start by converting the mcg to g as follows:

Method 1

Step 1, convert 9,000,000 mcg to mg by dividing by 1,000 as shown below

(9,000,000 micrograms /1,000) = 9,000 milligrams

Step 2, convert the 9,000 mg into g by dividing by 1,000

9,000 milligrams/1,000 = 9g

It therefore means that the required Ampicillin which was 9,000,000 mcg is the same as 9g.

If 20g of Ampicillin represents 1 tablet

9g of Ampicillin = ?

Cross multiplication as follows:

(9g/20g) x 1 tablet = 0.45 tablets

Method 2

We can also decide to change the 20g into mcg by considering the following.

1g = 1000 mg

Cross multiply as follows

$$\frac{20g}{1g} \times 1,000mg = 20,000mg$$

We can now convert the 20,000mg into mcg by multiplying by 1,000 as follows:

1mg = 1000mcg

20,000 mg = ?

Cross multiply as shown below

(20000 milligrams / 1mg) x 1,000 mcg = 20,000,000 micrograms (mcg)

This can now be interpreted as Ampicillin being available as 20,000,000 mcg tablets.

If 20,000,000 mcg Ampicillin represents 1 tablet

9,000,000 mcg Ampicillin = ?

Cross multiply as shown below

(9,000,000 micrograms/20,000,000 micrograms) = 0.45 tablets

The most important rule to note in such questions is ensuring that the values you are working with are in the same units.

The correct answer as proved by both methods is 0.45 tablets.

(103)  In this question you are required to calculate the amount of Solumedrolto be administered to a child who weighs 14 lb, if the doctor ordered 1.5 mg/kg and Solumedrol is available as 75 mg/ 1 mL.

We begin by making the units in the values similar.

We change the lb into kgs.

1lb = 0.4545 kg

14 lb = ?

We cross multiply as shown.

14 pounds / 1 pound x 0.4545 kilogram = 6.363 kilogram

Cross multiply as follows:

6.363kg/1kg x 1.5mg = 9.5445mg

We proceed and ask ourselves,

If 75mg of Solumedrol represents 1 mL

   9.5445mg of Solumedrol = ?

We cross multiply as shown:

9.5445 mg/75mg x 1ml = 0.1272ml

The correct answer is therefore 0.127mL.

(104)  In this question you are needed to calculate the amount of Sodium chloride in 1.5 L ½ NS.

It is important to note that NS is 0.9% Sodium Chloride

0.9 x ½ = 0.45%

Convert the L to mL

1L = 1,000mL

Cross multiply as follows

1.5l/1l x 1000ml = 1500ml

We finally use the formula

(Concentration % / 100) x volume in ml = Amount in grams

0.45/100 x 1500 = 6.75g

The correct answer is, therefore, 6.75g

(105)  Find out the quantity of sodium chloride contained in 1.5 liters ½ NS.

The correct answer for this question is 6.8 grams (g)

Workings

Here you will be calculating quantity contained in an IV fluid, and it is important to note that the concentration of sodium chloride in normal saline is always 0.9%.

½ x 0.9% = 0.45%

The formula for finding out the quantity of solid in a liquid is:

Percentrage in concentration/100 x Volume in milliliters (mL) = Dosage Quantity in grams (g)

Change the liters in the question to milliliters.

1.5 liters x 1,000 = 1,500 milliliters

(0.45% / 100) x 1,500 milliliters (mL) = 15 x 0.45% = 15 x 0.45 x (100/100) = 6.75

This can be rounded upwards to 6.8 grams (g)

(106)  The doctor has written a medication order for a child who weighs 15 pounds (lb). Calculate the rate of IV in terms of milliliters per hr (mL/hr) in order to ensure the right fluid level is maintained.

The right answer for this question is 28.41 milliliters per hour (mL/hr).

Workings

Since the appropriate fluid levels are provided in terms of patient's kilograms, it is important that the pounds be changed to metric, and the formula to change pounds to kilograms is dividing the given quantity by 2.2.

15 lb ÷ 2.2 = 6.81818 kg

This question on fluid maintenance requires the use of the schedule of kilogram ranges and the matching amount of fluids. A child whose weight is 6.81818 kg falls within the range of 0 kilograms to 10 kilograms, where you are supposed to provide 100 milliliters for every kilogram of the patient's weight.

6.81818 kg

6.81818 kg x 100 = 681.82 milliliters

You can now treat the problem as one of normal infusion of IV, where you use the formula:

Volume in milliliters / Time in hours = Rate of IV flow in milliliters per hour (mL/hr)

681.82 milliliters / 24hr = 28.41 milliliters per hour (mL/hr)

(107)  A medical practitioner has ordered that a child weighing 13 pounds be given the right amount of fluid each day. Calculate the appropriate amount in milliliters?

The right answer for this question is 590.91 milliliters (mL)

This is another question on fluid maintenance, one that requires you to remember the schedule of age category versus fluid levels.

13 pounds = (13 ÷ 2.2) kilograms = 5.909 kilograms

Again, this is a child whose weight falls within the range 0 kilograms to 10 kilograms, and where the fluid to be given is 100 milliliters per kilogram.

5.909 x 100 = 590.909 milliliters (mL)

(108)  The doctor ordered 0.00077 kiloliters (kL) D5W IV to be infused in a span of 15.6 hours using an infusion pump. Calculate the rate of IV flow in terms of milliliters per hour (mL/hr).

The right answer for this question is 49.4 milliliters per hour (mL/hr)

Workings

This is a question of volume per time versus the rate of IV flow, and the appropriate formula is

Volume in milliliters / Time in hours = Rate of IV flow in milliliters per hour (mL/hr)

You need to begin your workings by converting the kiloliters of fluid into milliliters, and the right way to do this is by multiplying the kiloliters by 1,000.

0.00077 kiloliters x 1,000 x 1,000 = 770 milliliters

The first conversion is to liters while the second conversion in sequence is to milliliters.

770 milliliters / 15.6 hours = 49.4 (mL/hr)

(109)  A young girl in the ward weighs 38 kilograms and the doctor has ordered that she be given enough fluid each day via IV. What should be the rate of IV flow in terms of milliliters per hour (mL/hr)?

The right answer for this question is 77.5 milliliters per hour (mL/hr).

Workings

The first step is to establish the amount of fluid the girl requires each day in order to maintain the appropriate fluid levels. For someone weighing 38 kilograms, the weight is within the range of 20 kilogram to 70 kilogram. The requirements for this range are 1,500 milliliters of fluid outright, and then additional 20 milliliters for every kilogram above the 20 kilogram mark. You can solve this problem through the equation:

Required milliliters = 1,500 + (38 − 20) x 20 = 1,500 + (18 x 20) = 1,500 + 360

Required milliliters = 1,860 milliliters (mL)

Now it is time to use the formula for IV rate given the fluid amount and time.

1,860 milliliters / 24hr = 77.7 (mL/hr)

(110)   The medical practitioner has ordered Potassium Chloride, as in the brand, K-Dur, and the amount in the order is 10,000,000 micrograms. However, from the hospital pharmacy, only 2 gram tablets are available. Calculate the number of tablets to be dispensed to the patient.

The right answer for this question is 5 tablets.

Workings

The formula that is helpful in a problem of this kind where the calculations involve mass versus mass is:

Quantity ordered / Quantity available = Number of tablets needed

First of all, it is necessary to convert 2 grams to micrograms, and to do this you need to multiply by 1,000 two times, the first time to get the milligrams and the second round to get the required micrograms.

2 x 1,000 x 1,000 = 2,000,000 micrograms (mcg)

10,000,000 / 2,000,000 = 5 tablets

(111)   The medical practitioner has ordered the drug, Solumedrol, 2.5 milligram per kilogram (mg/kg) and the prescription is for an infant who weighs just a kilogram, Considering the drug available at the pharmacy is in 125 milligrams per 2 milliliters (mg/ml), calculate the amount of fluid the nurse must administer to the infant.

The right answer for this question is 0.04 milliliters.

Workings

This question falls under the category of dosage by weight, and the appropriate formula to use first is:

Weight in kilograms x Dosage per kilogram = Needed Dosage

1 kilogram x 2.5 milligrams per kilogram = 2.5 milligrams

Then what follows is the formula to produce the amount of liquid needed, which is:

(Amount ordered / Amount available) x Volume per available = Liquid needed

(2.5 milligrams / 125 milligrams) x 2 milliliters = 0.04mL

(112)   The doctor has ordered 22 grams of Potassium Chloride, as in brand K-Dur, but the drug available is in tablets of 23,000,000 micrograms. How many of those tablets is the nurse supposed to dispense to the patient?

The right answer for this question is 1 tablet.

(Amount ordered / Amount available)= Number of tablets needed

Since the tablets to be dispensed are in micrograms, it is reasonable to convert the amount ordered to units of micrograms.

22 x 1,000 x 1,000 = 22,000,000 micrograms (mcg)

22,000,000 / 23,000,000 = 22/23 = 0.956, and this can be rounded to 1 tablet.

(113)   The doctor has prescribed Amoxicillin suspension for a one year old child who weighs 22 pound. The dosage for this child who has otitis media is 40 milligrams per kilogram per day, and it is divided BID. The hospital medication is packaged in concentrations of 400 milligrams per 5 milliliters.

Find out the Amoxicillin dose in terms of milliliters.

The answer for this question is 2.5 milliliters BID.

Workings

Begin by converting pounds to kilograms. This will work out like this:

22 pounds x 1 kilogram per 2.2 pounds or simply 22 ÷ 2.2, and this becomes 10 kilograms.

The next step is to find out the dose in milligrams, and the way to do this is:

10 kilograms x 40 milligrams per kilogram per day, and this works to 400 milligrams per day.

In the 3rd step, you need to divide the exact dose by the prescribed frequency. Frequency is represented by BID, which is simply 2 time a day, so:

400 milligrams per day ÷ 2 = 200 milligrams per dose BID

The last step involves converting the milligram dose to milliliters as follows:

200 milligrams per dose ÷ 400 milligrams per 5 milliliters = 2.5 milliliters BID

(114)   The medical practitioner has prescribed ceftriaxone for a child whose weight is 18 kilograms. This dose, which is meant to treat meningitis, is 100 milligram per kilogram per day, and it is to be administered in IV. The drug comes to the hospital pre-diluted, and it is in a concentration of 40 milligrams per milliliter. Calculate the dosage the nurse is supposed to administer in milliliters.

The answer for this question is 45 milliliters once in a day.

Workings

The first step is to do calculations that will give you the dose in milligrams like this:

18 kilograms x 100 milligrams per kilograms per day = 1,800 milligrams per day

The next step is dividing that dose based on the frequency it should be administered like this:

1800 milligrams per day ÷ 1 = 1,800 milligrams per dose

In step three, you need to convert the milligram dose to milliliters as follows:

1,800 milligrams per dose ÷ 40 milligrams per milliliter = 45 milliliter once a day

(115)   In this question, you are required to calculate the flow rate in mL/hr in which you are going to set an IV pump in order to administer a bolus dose of 60 units / kg to a patient who weighs 198 lbs. The doctor orders that the Heparin IV drip starts at 16units/kg and you are offered with a Heparin bag that reads 12,500 units/ 250mL.

The correct answer for this question is therefore, 28.797mL/hr

Workings

Start by converting the weight in lbs to kgs.

This is done by considering that:

   1 lb  = 0.4545kgs

We cross multiply as shown below

0.4545 kilogram / 1 pound x 198 pounds = 89.991 kilograms

We proceed and ask ourselves,

If      1 kg represents 16 units

16 units kilograms per hour / 1 kilogram x 89.991 kilograms = 1,439.856 units per hr

This simply means that if the doctor ordered that the patient is administered with Heparin at 16 units/kg/hr and our patient weighs 89.991 kgs, then the patient will require 1439.856 units of Heparin. We will now need to calculate the flow rate in mL/hr in which the pump will have to be set at.

If

12500 units = 250 ml

We cross multiply as shown below:

250ml / 12,500 units x 1,439.856 units/hr = 28.797

(116)   In this question we are required to find out the number of units a patient is receiving per hour if the Heparin drip is running at 36 mL/hr and the Heparin bag reads 12,500 units/ 250 mL.

The correct answer for this question is therefore, 1,800 units / hr.

<u>Workings</u>

We start by understanding the relationship between the various values in the question as follows:

If per every 250 mL the patient receives 12,500 units, then how many units does the patient receive if 36 mL of Heparin is administered per hour?

The above statement can be interpreted as follows:

250 mL = 12,500 units

Cross multiply as shown below:

12500 units /250 milliliters x 36 milliliters / hour = 1800 units / hour

(117)   In this question we are tasked with calculating the amount of Heparin a patient receives per hour if the Heparin drip is running at 29 mL/hr and the Heparin bag reads 10,000 units/ 100 mL.

The correct answer for this question is 2,900 units / hr

<u>Workings</u>

It is important to start by understanding and interpreting the question correctly as follows:

If per every 100 mL of medicine administered there are 10,000 units of Heparin, then how many units of Heparin are administered in 29 mL of medicine?

The above statement can be written as follows:

100 mL = 10,000 units

Cross multiply as follows:

10,000 units / 100 milliliters x 29 milliliters / hour = 2,900 units / hour

(118)  We are required to calculate the flow rate in mL/hr, for a patient who weighs 129 lbs. The drip starts at 24 units/kgs/hr and the Heparin bags reads 25,000 units/250 mL.

The correct answer is 14.07132 mL/hr.

<u>Workings</u>

We start by converting 129 lbs to kgs by considering the following relationship,

1 lb = 0.4545 kg

Cross multiply:

0.4545 kilograms / 1 pound x 129 pounds = 58.63 kilograms

If 1 kg represents 24 units

Cross multiply

24 units / kilogram x 58.63 kilograms = 1,407 units

We complete by asking ourselves, if 25,000 units are found in 250 mL, then 1,407 units will be found in how many mL?

The above statement can be written as follows:

25,000 units  means 250 Ml

Cross multiply as follows:

250    lliliters / 25,000 units x 1,407 units = 14 milliliters / hour

(119) The medication order indicates the patient, who is a boy with leukemia aged 4yrs, requires the drug, vincristine. The boy weighs 37 pounds and happens to be 97 centimeters in height. The order indicates a dose of 2 milligrams per square meter but the drug at the hospital is in dosage of 1 milligram per milliliter.

Find out the vincristine dose to be dispensed in milliliters.

The correct answer for this question is 1.34 milliliters (mL).

Workings

Begin by converting pounds to kilograms as follows:

37 pounds x 1 kilogram per 2.2 pounds = 16.8 kilograms

Next, find the BSA as shown below:

$\sqrt{}$16.8 kilograms x 97 centimeters per 3,600 = 0.67m²

The step to follow next is calculating the dose in milligrams as follows:

2 milligrams per m² x 0.67 m²  = 1.34 milligrams

Finally you need to find out the dose this time in milliliters as shown below:

1.34 milligrams ÷ 1  milligram per milliliter = 1.34 milliliter.

(120)  The doctor has prescribed 4 tablets of the medication, Z, and the patient is to take it two times a day, 6/7. How many should the nurse dispense to the patient for the full dose?

The right answer for this question is 48 tablets.

Workings

The order of 4 tablets two times a day, means in a day the number will be:

4 tablets x 2 = 8 tablets

6/7 simply means 6 days in the week, so it means on the whole the patient needs to take: 8 tablets x 6, which results to 48 tablets.

(121) The physician has prescribed a patient 15 milliliters of cough medication, to take 4 times each day for seven days. How many doses should the patient be given?

The right answer for this question is 28 doses.

If one day = 4 doses, how many doses will there be in 7 days?

7 days = 4 doses x 7, which results to 28 doses.

www.ingramcontent.com/pod-product-compliance
Lightning Source LLC
Chambersburg PA
CBHW060926210326
41597CB00042B/4515